# Virtual Medical Office

for

## Young: Kinn's The Administrative Medical Assistant, 6th Edition

# Virtual Medical Office

for

# Young: Kinn's The Administrative Medical Assistant, 6th Edition

*Study Guide prepared by*

**Eugenia M. Fulcher, RN, BSN, EdD, CMA**

Formerly
Instructor and Program Director, Medical Assisting and Nursing
Swainsboro Technical College
Swainsboro, Georgia

Instructor, Nursing
University Hospital School of Nursing
Augusta, Georgia

Nursing Supervisor and Office Manager
Dr. Charles Green
Waynesboro, Georgia

*Textbook by*

**Alexandra Patricia Young, BBA, RMA, CMA**

Professional Writer
Irving, Texas

Formerly
Director of Admissions
Parker College of Chiropractic
Dallas, Texas

Formerly
Program Director
Medical Assisting/HIM Programs
Ultrasound Diagnostic School
Irving, Texas

*software developed by*

**Wolfsong Informatics, LLC**
Tucson, Arizona

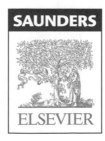

SAUNDERS

ELSEVIER

# SAUNDERS
ELSEVIER

11830 Westline Industrial Dr.
St. Louis, Missouri 63146

VIRTUAL MEDICAL OFFICE FOR
YOUNG: KINN'S THE ADMINISTRATIVE MEDICAL ASSISTANT
SIXTH EDITION
**Copyright © 2007 by Saunders, an imprint of Elsevier Inc.**

ISBN: 978-1-4160-4186-3

Although for mechanical reasons all pages of this publication are perforated, only those pages
imprinted with an Elsevier Inc. copyright notice are intended for removal.

---

### Notice

Knowledge and best practice in this field are constantly changing. As new research and experience
broaden our knowledge, changes in practice, treatment and drug therapy may become necessary or
appropriate. Readers are advised to check the most current information provided (i) on procedures
featured or (ii) by the manufacturer of each product to be administered, to verify the recommended
dose or formula, the method and duration of administration, and contraindications. It is the
responsibility of the practitioner, relying on their own experience and knowledge of the patient, to
make diagnoses, to determine dosages and the best treatment for each individual patient, and to
take all appropriate safety precautions. To the fullest extent of the law, neither the Publisher nor
the Authors assumes any liability for any injury and/or damage to persons or property arising out
or related to any use of the material contained in this book.

---

ISBN: 978-1-4160-4186-3

*Acquisitions Editor:* Susan Cole
*Managing Editor:* Scott Weaver
*Senior Developmental Editor:* Donna Morrissey
*Publishing Services Manager:* Linda McKinley
*Project Manager:* Stephen Bancroft
*Cover Designer:* Mark Oberkrom

Printed in the United States of America

Last digit is the print number: 9 8 7 6 5 4 3 2 1

Working together to grow
libraries in developing countries

www.elsevier.com | www.bookaid.org | www.sabre.org

ELSEVIER    BOOK AID International    Sabre Foundation

# Table of Contents

## Reviewers

**Susanna M. Hancock, AAS, RMA, CMA, RPT, COLT**
American Medical Technologist Board Member
ABHES, School Evaluator
Former Medical Assistant Director
American Institute of Health Technology
Boise, Idaho

**Rebecca Hickey, RN, RMC, AHI, CHI**
Butler Technology and Career Development Schools
Fairfield Township, Ohio

**Sue A. Hunt, MA, RN, CMA**
Professor and Coordinator of Medical Assisting
Middlesex Community College
Lowell, Massachusetts

# Getting Started

## GETTING SET UP

### ■ RECOMMENDED SYSTEM REQUIREMENTS

#### WINDOWS™

Windows® PC
Windows XP
Pentium® processor (or equivalent) @ 1 GHz (Recommend 2 GHz or better)
1.5 GB hard disk space
512 MB of RAM (Recommend 1 GB or more)
CD-ROM drive
800 x 600 screen size
Thousands of colors
Soundblaster 16 soundcard compatibility
Stereo speakers or headphones

#### MACINTOSH®

*Virtual Medical Office* is not compatible with the Macintosh platform.

### ■ INSTALLATION INSTRUCTIONS

#### WINDOWS

1. Insert the *Virtual Medical Office* CD-ROM.
2. Inserting the CD should automatically bring up the setup screen if the current product is not already installed.
   a. If the setup screen does not appear automatically (and *Virtual Medical Office* has not been installed already), navigate to the "My Computer" icon on your desktop or in your Start menu.
   b. Double-click on your CD-ROM drive.
   c. If installation does not start at this point:
      (1) Click the **Start** icon on the task bar and select the **Run** option.
      (2) Type d:\setup.exe (where "d:\" is your CD-ROM drive) and press **OK**.
      (3) Follow the onscreen instructions for installation.
3. Follow the onscreen instructions during the setup process.

## ■ HOW TO LAUNCH VIRTUAL MEDICAL OFFICE

### WINDOWS

1. Double-click on the *Virtual Medical Office* icon located on your desktop.
2. Or navigate to the program via the Windows Start menu.


## ■ SCREEN SETTINGS

For best results, your computer monitor resolution should be set at a minimum of 800 x 600. The number of colors displayed should be set to "thousands or higher" (High Color or 16 bit) or "millions of colors" (True Color or 24 bit).

### WINDOWS

1. From the **Start** menu, select **Settings**, then **Control Panel**.
2. Double-click on the **Display** icon.
3. Click on the **Settings** tab.
4. Under **Screen resolution** use the slider bar to select **800 by 600 pixels**.
5. Access the **Colors** drop-down menu by clicking on the down arrow.
6. Select **High Color (16 bit)** or **True Color (24 bit)**.
7. Click on **OK**.
8. You may be asked to verify the setting changes. Click **Yes**.
9. You may be asked to restart your computer to accept the changes. Click **Yes**.


## ■ TECHNICAL SUPPORT

Technical support for this product is available between 7:30 a.m. and 7 p.m. (CST), Monday through Friday. Before calling, be sure that your computer meets the system requirements to run this software. Inside the United States and Canada, call 1-800-692-9010. Outside North America, call 314-872-8370. You may also fax your questions to 314-523-4932 or contact Technical Support through e-mail: technical.support@elsevier.com.

Trademarks: Windows, Pentium, and America Online are registered trademarks.

Copyright © 2007 by Saunders, an imprint of Elsevier Inc.

# ACCESSING *Virtual Medical Office Online Study Guide* ON EVOLVE

The product you have purchased is part of the Evolve family of online courses and learning resources. Please read the following information thoroughly to get started.

**To access the *Virtual Medical Office Online Study Guide* on Evolve:**

Your instructor will provide you with the username and password needed to access the *Virtual Medical Office Online Study Guide* on the Evolve Learning System. Once you have received this information, please follow these instructions:

1. Go to the Evolve login page (http://evolve.elsevier.com/login)

2. Enter your username and password in the **Login to My Evolve** area and click the arrow or hit **Enter**.

3. You will be taken to your personalized **My Evolve** page, where the course will be listed in the **My Courses** module.

## TECHNICAL REQUIREMENTS

To use the *Virtual Medical Office Online Study Guide*, you will need access to a computer that is connected to the Internet and equipped with web browser software that supports frames. For optimal performance, it is recommended that you have speakers and use a high-speed Internet connection. However, slower dial-up modems (56 K minimum) are acceptable.

## ■ WEB BROWSERS

Supported web browsers include Microsoft Internet Explorer (IE) version 6.0 or higher, Netscape version 7.1 or higher, and Mozilla Firefox version 1.4 or higher.

If you use America Online (AOL) for web access, you will need AOL version 4.0 or higher and IE 5.0 or higher. Do not use earlier versions of AOL with earlier versions of IE, because you will have difficulty accessing many features.

For best results with AOL:
- Connect to the Internet using AOL version 4.0 or higher.
- Open a private chat within AOL (this allows the AOL client to remain open, without asking whether you wish to disconnect while minimized).
- Minimize AOL.
- Launch a recommended browser.

Whichever browser you use, the browser preferences must be set to enable cookies and JavaScript and the cache must be set to reload every time.

## Enable Cookies

| Browser | Steps |
|---|---|
| Internet Explorer (IE) 6.0 or higher | 1. Select **Tools → Internet Options**. <br> 2. Select **Privacy** tab. <br> 3. Use the slider (slide down) to **Accept All Cookies**. <br> 4. Click **OK**. <br><br> -OR- <br><br> 3. Click the **Advanced** button. <br> 4. Click the check box next to **Override Automatic Cookie Handling**. <br> 5. Click the **Accept** radio buttons under **First-party Cookies** and **Third-party Cookies**. <br> 6. Click **OK**. |
| Netscape 7.1 or higher | 1. Select **Edit → Preferences**. <br> 2. Select **Privacy & Security**. <br> 3. Select **Cookies**. <br> 4. Select **Enable All Cookies**. |
| Mozilla Firefox 1.4 or higher | 1. Select **Tools → Options**. <br> 2. Select the **Privacy** icon. <br> 3. Click to expand Cookies. <br> 4. Select **Allow sites to set cookies**. <br> 5. Click **OK**. |

## Enable JavaScript

| Browser | Steps |
|---|---|
| Internet Explorer (IE) 6.0 or higher | 1. Select **Tools → Internet Options**.<br>2. Select **Security** tab.<br>3. Under **Security level for this zone** set to **Medium** or lower. |
| Netscape 7.1 or higher | 1. Select **Edit → Preferences**.<br>2. Select **Advanced**.<br>3. Select **Scripts & Plugins**.<br>4. Make sure the **Navigator** box is checked to **Enable JavaScript**.<br>5. Click **OK**. |
| Mozilla Firefox 1.4 or higher | 1. Select **Tools → Options**.<br>2. Select the **Content** icon.<br>3. Select **Enable JavaScript**.<br>4. Click **OK**. |

## Set Cache to Always Reload a Page

| Browser | Steps |
|---|---|
| Internet Explorer (IE) 6.0 or higher | 1. Select **Tools → Internet Options**.<br>2. Select **General** tab.<br>3. Go to the **Temporary Internet Files** and click the **Settings** button.<br>4. Select the radio button for **Every visit to the page** and click **OK** when complete. |
| Netscape 7.1 or higher | 1. Select **Edit → Preferences**.<br>2. Select **Advanced**.<br>3. Select **Cache**.<br>4. Select the **Every time I view the page** radio button.<br>5. Click **OK**. |
| Mozilla Firefox 1.4 or higher | 1. Select **Tools → Options**.<br>2. Select the **Privacy** icon.<br>3. Click to expand Cache.<br>4. Set the value to "0" in the **Use up to: __ MB of disk space for the cache** field.<br>5. Click **OK**. |

## Plug-Ins

**Adobe Acrobat Reader**—With the free Acrobat Reader software, you can view and print Adobe PDF files. Many Evolve products offer student and instructor manuals, checklists, and more in this format!

**Download at:** http://www.adobe.com

**Apple QuickTime**—Install this to hear word pronunciations, heart and lung sounds, and many other helpful audio clips within Evolve Online Courses!

**Download at:** http://www.apple.com

**Adobe Flash Player**—This player will enhance your viewing of many Evolve web pages, as well as educational short-form to long-form animation within the Evolve Learning System!

**Download at:** http://www.adobe.com

**Adobe Shockwave Player**—Shockwave is best for viewing the many interactive learning activities within Evolve Online Courses!

**Download at:** http://www.adobe.com

**Microsoft Word Viewer**—With this viewer Microsoft Word users can share documents with those who don't have Word, and users without Word can open and view Word documents. Many Evolve products have testbank, student and instructor manuals, and other documents available for downloading and viewing on your own computer!

**Download at:** http://www.microsoft.com

**Microsoft PowerPoint Viewer**—View PowerPoint 97, 2000, and 2002 presentations even if you don't have PowerPoint with this viewer. Many Evolve products have slides available for downloading and viewing on your own computer!

**Download at:** http://www.microsoft.com

## SUPPORT INFORMATION

**Live support** is available to customers in the United States and Canada from 7:30 a.m. to 7 p.m. (CST), Monday through Friday by calling **1-800-401-9962**. You can also send an email to evolve-support@elsevier.com.

There is also **24/7 support information** available on the Evolve website (http://evolve.elsevier.com), including:

- Guided Tours
- Tutorials
- Frequently Asked Questions (FAQs)
- Online Copies of Course User Guides
- And much more!

# Office Tour

Welcome to *Virtual Medical Office*, a virtual office setting in which you can work with multiple patient simulations and also learn to access and evaluate the information resources that are essential for providing high-quality medical assistance.

In the virtual medical office, Mountain View Clinic, you can access the Reception area, Exam Room, Laboratory, Office Manager, and Check-Out area, plus a separate room for Billing and Coding.

## ■ BEFORE YOU START

Make sure you have your textbook nearby when you use the *Virtual Medical Office* CD. You will want to consult topic areas in your textbook frequently while working with the CD and using this study guide.

## ■ HOW TO SIGN IN

- Double-click on the *Virtual Medical Office* icon on your computer's desktop to start the program.
- Once the software has loaded, enter your name on the Medical Assistant identification badge
- Click on **Start Simulation**.

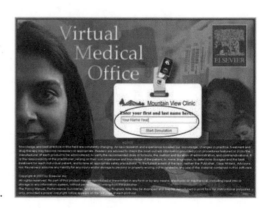

*Enter your name and click Start Simulation.*

- This takes you to the office map screen. Across the top of this screen is the list of patients available for you to follow throughout their office visit.

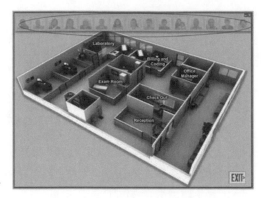

*Office map with patient list.*

## ■ PATIENT LIST

1. **Janet Jones (age 50)**—Ms. Jones has sustained an on-the-job injury. She is in pain and impatient. By working with Ms. Jones, students will learn about managing difficult patients, as well as the requirements involved in Workers' Compensation cases.

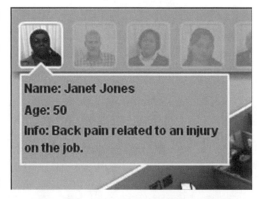

*Janet Jones*

2. **Wilson Metcalf (age 65)**—A Medicare patient, Mr. Metcalf is being seen for multiple symptoms of abdominal pain, nausea, vomiting, and fever. He is seriously ill and might need more specialized care in a hospital setting.

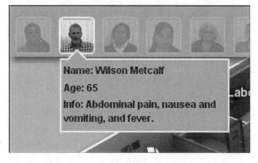

*Wilson Metcalf*

3. **Rhea Davison (age 53)**—An established patient with chronic and multiple symptoms, Ms. Davison does not have medical insurance.

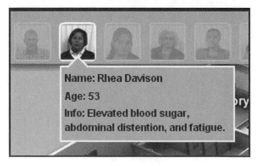

*Rhea Davison*

4. **Shaunti Begay (age 15)**—A new patient, Shaunti Begay is a minor who has an appointment for a sports physical. Upon arrival, Shaunti and her family learn that Mountain View Clinic does not participate in their health insurance.

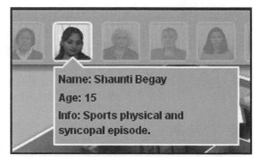

*Shaunti Begay*

5. **Jean Deere (age 83)**—Accompanied by her son, Ms. Deere is an established Medicare patient being evaluated for memory loss and hearing loss.

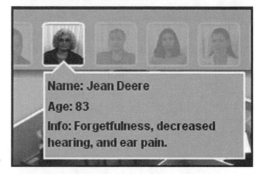

*Jean Deere*

6. **Renee Anderson (age 43)**—Ms. Anderson scheduled her appointment for a routine gynecologic exam but exhibits symptoms that suggest she is a victim of domestic violence.

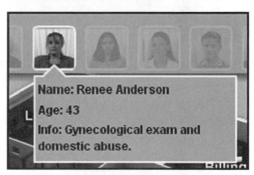

*Renee Anderson*

7. **Teresa Hernandez (age 16)**—Teresa is a minor patient who is unaccompanied by a parent for her appointment. She is seeking contraceptive counseling and STD testing.

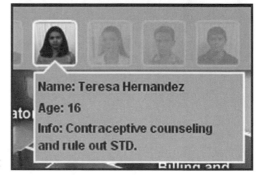

*Teresa Hernandez*

8. **Louise Parlet (age 24)**—Ms. Parlet is an established patient being seen for a pregnancy test and examination. She will also need to be referred to an OB/GYN specialist.

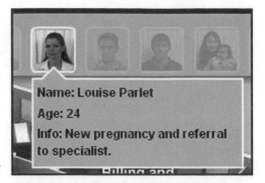

*Louise Parlet*

9. **Tristan Tsosie (age 8)**—A minor patient accompanied by his older sister and younger brother, Tristan is having a splint and sutures removed from his injured right arm.

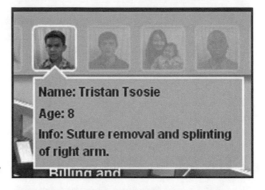

*Tristan Tsosie*

10. **Jose Imero (age 16)**—Jose is a minor patient who is scheduled for an emergency appointment to have the laceration on his foot sutured.

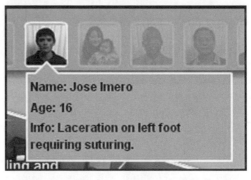

*Jose Imero*

11. **Jade Wong (age 7 months)**—Jade and her parents are new patients to Mountain View Clinic. Jade needs a checkup and updates to her immunizations. Her mother does not speak English.

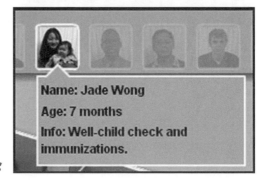

*Jade Wong*

12. **John R. Simmons (age 43)**—Dr. Simmons is a new patient with a history of high blood pressure and recent episodes of blood in his urine.

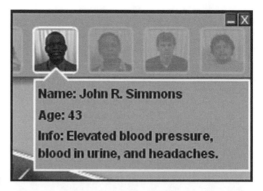

*John R. Simmons*

13. **Hu Huang (age 67)**—Mr. Huang developed a severe cough and fever after returning from a recent trip to Asia.

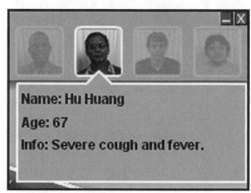

*Hu Huang*

14. **Kevin McKinzie (age 18)**—Mr. McKinzie has made an appointment because of his nausea and vomiting. He is insured through the restaurant where he works.

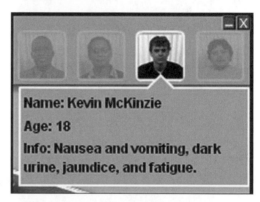

*Kevin McKinzie*

15. **Jesus Santo (age 32)**—Mr. Santo has been brought to the office as a walk-in appointment by his employer for leg pain and a fever. He has no insurance or identification, but his employer has offered to pay for the visit.

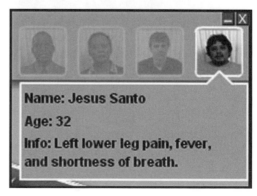

*Jesus Santo*

## ■ BASIC NAVIGATION

### HOW TO SELECT A PATIENT

The list of patients is located across the top of the office map screen. Pointing your cursor at the various patients will highlight their photo and reveal their name, age, and medical problem (see examples in the photos on the previous pages). When you click on the patient you wish to review, a larger photo and description will appear in the lower left corner of the screen.

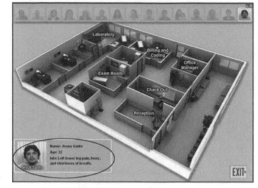

*Click on a photo to select a patient.*

*Note:* You **must** select a patient before you are allowed access to the Reception area, Exam Room, Laboratory, Billing and Coding office, or Check Out area. The Office Manager area is the only room you can enter without first selecting a patient.

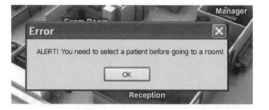

*Select a patient before choosing a room.*

### HOW TO SELECT A ROOM

After selecting a patient, use your cursor to highlight the room you want to enter. The active room will be shaded blue on the map. Click to enter the room.

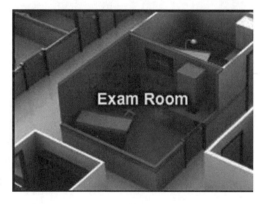

*Highlight and click on a room to enter.*

### HOW TO LEAVE A ROOM

When you are finished working in a room, you can leave by clicking the exit arrow found at the bottom right corner of the screen.

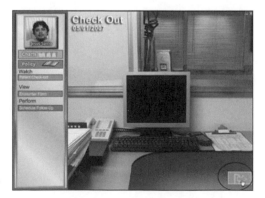

*Click on the exit arrow.*

Leaving a room will automatically take you to the Summary Menu.

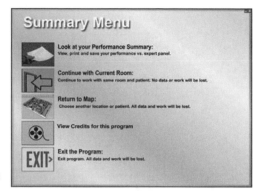

*The Summary Menu*

From the Summary Menu, you can choose to:

- **Look at Your Performance Summary**

    In each room there are interactive wizards or tasks that can be completed. The Performance Summary lets you compare your answers with those of the experts.

- **Continue with Current Room**

    This takes you back to the last room in which you worked. This option is not available if you have already reviewed your Performance Summary.

- **Return to Map**

    This reopens the office map for you to select another room and/or another patient.

- **View Credits for This Program**

    This provides a complete listing of software developers, publisher, and authors.

- **Exit the Program**

    This closes the *Virtual Medical Office* software. You will need to sign in again before you can use the program.

### HOW TO USE THE PERFORMANCE SUMMARY

If you completed any of the interactive wizards in a room, you can compare your answers with those of the experts by accessing your Performance Summary. The Performance Summary is not a grading tool, although it is valuable for self-assessment and review.

From the Summary Menu, click on **Look at Your Performance Summary**.

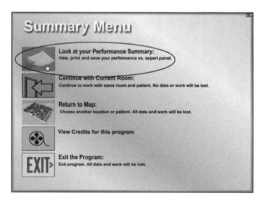

*Select Look at Your Performance Summary.*

The complete list of tasks associated with the active room will appear with two columns showing the results of your choices. Your answers will appear in the column labeled **Your Performance**, and the answers chosen by the expert will appear in the **Expert's Performance** column. A check mark in the same box in both columns indicates that your answer matched the expert's answer. The Performance Summary can be saved to your computer or disk by clicking on the disk icon at the upper right side of the screen. The saved file can be printed or e-mailed to your instructor. A hard copy can also be printed without saving by clicking on the printer icon at the upper right corner of the screen.

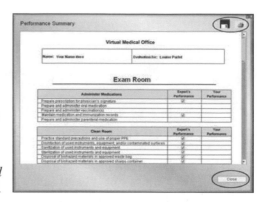

*The Performance Summary can be printed and/or saved.*

## ■ ROOM DESCRIPTIONS

Each room can be entered at any time in any order. You can follow a patient's visit from Reception to Check Out, or you can choose to observe each patient at any point in their care. Below is a description of the information and activities that can be found in various rooms.

### ALL ROOMS

- In all rooms you can access the patient's medical record and the office Policy Manual.

- In all rooms in which there are interactive tasks to be completed, you can select tasks or features from the menu on the left of the screen, as shown on this sample of the menu in the Reception area.

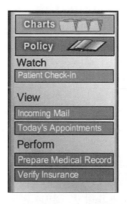

*Reception area menu*

- As an alternative to using the menu, you can click on the corresponding items in the photo of the room. As you move your cursor over each item connected to one of the tasks on the menu, it will highlight and become active.

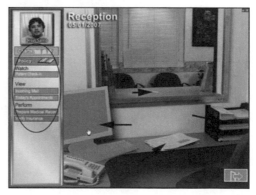

*Reception area*

## RECEPTION

In the Reception area, you can choose:

- **Charts**—Look at the patient's chart. *Note:* For new patients, there will be no information available in the chart at this time although you do have the option of assembling a new medical record.
- **Policy**—Open the office Policy Manual and review the established administrative, clinical, and laboratory policies for Mountain View Clinic. Within the Policy Manual you will also find the Coding and Billing Manual.
- **Watch**—Watch a video of the patient's arrival. Each patient is shown checking in at the front desk so that you can observe the procedures typically performed by the receptionist and consider some of the various problems that might arise.
- **Incoming Mail**—Look at the incoming mail for the day. Mountain View Clinic has received a wide range of correspondence that must be read and responded to accordingly.
- **Today's Appointments**—Review the appointment schedule for the day. You can check the schedule to find out what time patients are supposed to arrive, the reason for their visit, and how much time the physician will need for the examination.
- **Prepare Medical Record**—Practice preparing the medical record. This interactive feature allows you to build a medical record for a new patient or update information for an established patient.
- **Verify Insurance**—Verify a patient's insurance. Also interactive, this feature allows you to ask patients about the status of their insurance and to view their insurance cards.

## EXAM ROOM

- **Charts** and **Policy**—Access the patient's chart and the office Policy Manual.
- **Watch**—View video clips of different parts of the patient's exam. Observe the actions of the medical assistants in the videos and critique the competencies demonstrated.
- **Exam Notes**—Review the physician's documented findings for the current visit. These notes are added to the full Progress Notes in the patient's chart as the patient continues on to Check Out.
- **Perform**—Perform multiple tasks that are required of a clinical medical assistant, such as preparing the room for the exam, taking vital signs and patient history, and properly positioning the patient for an exam.

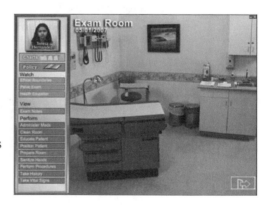

### LABORATORY

- **Charts** and **Policy**—Access the patient's chart and the office Policy Manual.
- **View: Logs**—View the laboratory's log of specimens sent out for testing. Opportunities to practice filling out laboratory logs are included in the workbook exercises.
- **Perform**—Perform specific tasks as needed in the laboratory, such as collecting and testing specimens. These interactive wizards walk you through the steps for collecting and testing specimens ordered by the physician as part of the patient's examination. The Progress Notes are available throughout so that you can review the physician's directions.

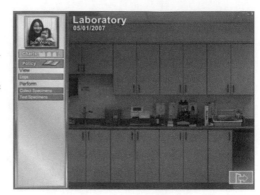

### CHECK OUT

- **Charts** and **Policy**—Access the patient's chart and the office Policy Manual.
- **Watch**—Watch a video clip of the patient checking out of the office at the end of the visit. Observe the administrative medical assistants as they schedule follow-up appointments, accept payments, and manage the various duties and problems that may arise.
- **View**—Look at the Encounter Form completed for each patient and verify that the form is filled out correctly and completely.
- **Perform**—Certain patients will require a return visit to the office. Schedule their follow-up appointments as needed. Opportunities to work with the appointment book and additional scheduling tasks are included in the study guide.

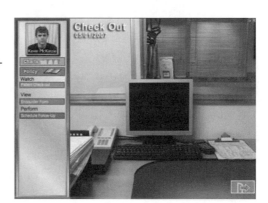

### BILLING AND CODING

- **View: Aging Report**—Review the outstanding balances on various patient accounts and assess when to implement different collection techniques.
- **View: Encounter Form**—Review the patient's Encounter Form and determine whether the proper procedures were followed to ensure accurate billing and coding.
- **View: Fee Schedule**—Review the office's fee schedule to calculate the proper charges for the patient's visit.

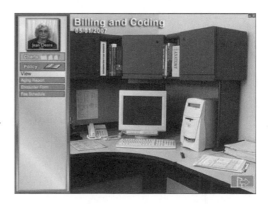

### OFFICE MANAGER

- **Policy**—View the office Policy Manual. Note that patient charts are not available from the manager's office, and there is no need to select a patient to enter the Office Manager area.
- **View**—A variety of financial and administrative documents are available for viewing in the manager's office. Banking deposits and payments can be tracked through these documents, and opportunities to practice managing office finances are included in the study guide.
- **Perform: Transcribe Report**—A recorded medical report is included for transcription practice with full player controls.

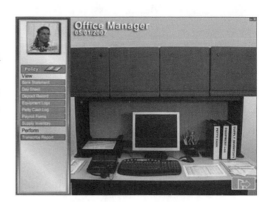

## ■ EMBEDDED ERRORS

The individual lessons and patient scenarios associated with the *Virtual Medical Office* program were designed to stimulate critical thinking and analytical skills and to help develop the competencies you will be tested on as part of your course work. Thus deliberate errors have been embedded into each of the 15 patient scenarios and in the Billing and Coding and Office Manager activities. Many of the exercises in the study guide draw attention to these errors so that you can work through how and why a correction needs to be made. Other errors have not been specifically addressed, and you may discover them as you work through the various rooms and tasks. Instructors and students alike are encouraged to use any errors they find to further develop the essential critical thinking and decision-making skills needed for the clinical office.

The following icons are used throughout the study guide to help you quickly identify particular activities and assignments:

 Reading Assignment—tells you which textbook chapter(s) you should read before starting each lesson

 Writing Activity—certain activities focus on written responses such as filling out forms or completing documentation

 CD-ROM Activity—marks the beginning of an activity that uses the *Virtual Medical Office* simulation software

 CD-ROM Instructions—indicates the steps to follow as you navigate through the software

 Reference—indicates questions and activities that require you to consult your textbook

 Time—indicates the approximate amount of time needed to complete the exercise

# Performing Other Professional Duties

∞ **Reading Assignment:** Chapter 3—The Medical Assisting Profession
    • Professional Appearance
Chapter 4—Professional Behavior in the Workplace
Chapter 5—Interpersonal Skills and Human Behavior

**Patient:** Rhea Davison

**Objectives:**

- Prepare the documentation for possible termination of patient.
- Describe the necessary documentation of licensure and accreditation.
- Recognize the need for confidentiality and HIPPA regulations.
- Prepare a travel itinerary for a physician in the medical office.
- Locate resources and information for the employer.
- Describe the need for and the maintenance of liability coverage.

**Overview:**

In this lesson you will prepare documentation needed for assisting the physician in various areas related to office policies and the physician's professional needs. The ethical and legal aspects of confidentiality are addressed, as well as how to deal with patients who habitually cancel appointments. The Internet will be used to research travel arrangements for a conference one of the physicians needs to attend. Finally, the importance of maintaining liability insurance will be discussed.

### Exercise 1

## CD-ROM Activity—Recognizing the Need for Patient Termination

30 minutes

- Sign in to Mountain View Clinic.
- Select Rhea Davison from the patient list and click on **Reception**.

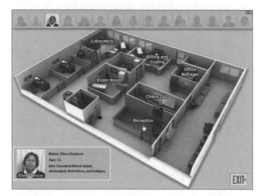

*Click on Reception.*

- At the Reception desk, click on **Today's Appointments** to review the day's schedule.

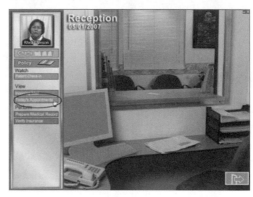

*Click on Today's Appointments.*

1. Who is the patient who has canceled an appointment, and what was the patient's chief complaint?

2. What is the role of the medical assistant in providing information about cancellations to the physician?

- When you obtain the medical record to document the cancellation, you discover that this patient has canceled and rescheduled this appointment three times. He is now 4 weeks late for a return appointment.
- Click **Finish** to close the appointment book and return to the Reception desk.
- Click on **Policy** to open the office Policy Manual.

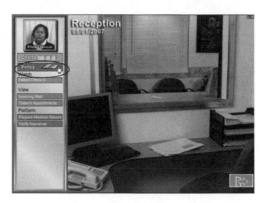

*Click on Policy.*

- Type "cancel" in the search bar and click the magnifying glass once to read the office policy regarding canceled appointments.
- Click **Close Manual** to return to the Reception desk.

3. According to the Policy Manual, what is the next step to be taken with this patient who has canceled his last three appointments? Explain your answer.

4. Below, compose a letter to the patient you identified in question 2. In the letter, describe the reason for possible termination and the necessary steps needed to remain a patient of Dr. Meyer. The letter should include all of the reasons for possible termination and the need for the patient to keep appointments as made. The letter can also state that Dr. Meyer is concerned about continuity of care and the need for patient safety through this continuity of care.

**Mountain View Clinic**

4412 Broadway / London, XY 55555 / Phone: (555) 555-1234 / Fax (555) 555-1239

*Nathan Hayler, MD - Family Practice / Katarina Meyer, MD - Internal Medicine*

5. Why does the letter need to be certified?

6. If a decision is made to terminate a patient, how much time must be allowed between notification and the termination?

 • Remain in the Reception area with Rhea Davison and continue to the next exercise.

### Exercise 2

 **CD-ROM Activity—Maintaining Licensure and Credentials**

 15 minutes

• At the Reception desk with Rhea Davison, click on **Patient Check-In** to view the video. (*Note:* If you have exited the program, sign in again to Mountain View Clinic, select Rhea Davison from the patient list, go to the Reception area, and view the video.)
• At the end of the video, click **Close**.

1. In the video, the medical assistant discusses the CMA credential. However, the RMA is another credential that is recognized on a national level. What does RMA mean, and what is the accrediting agency?

2. On arrival this morning, Dr. Meyer states that you need to check on the status of her renewed medical license because it has not arrived. She reminds you that her current license expires on June 1. Go to the Internet and find the name and address of the medical examining board for the state in which you live. Also find the time limit for medical licensure and any necessary components for renewal of the license. Print your findings for your instructor.

 • Remain in the Reception area and continue to the next exercise.

**Exercise 3**

 **CD-ROM Activity—Maintaining Confidentiality and Explaining Office Policy to the Patient**

 30 minutes

- This exercise continues with questions regarding the video of Rhea Davison's check-in. If you need to review the video again, click on **Patient Check-In** at the Reception desk. (*Note:* If you have exited the program, sign in again to Mountain View Clinic, select Rhea Davison from the patient list, go to the Reception area, and view the video again if necessary.)

  1. Ms. Davison is an established patient. Did Kristin handle Ms. Davison's lateness in a professional manner? Explain your answer.

  2. What was your feeling about Kristin and the issue of confidentiality just before the arrival of the office manager?

  3. The office manager explained the need to follow HIPPA policy and the need for confidentiality of medical records. How do you feel about the attitude of the office manager while discussing the matter of confidentiality?

  4. Why does the office manager need to explain HIPPA policy in such a specific manner?

**Exercise 4**

 **Writing Activity—Obtaining Travel Itineraries and Locating Information for the Physician**

 30 minutes

1. Prepare and provide a travel itinerary for one of the physicians at Mountain View Clinic, following these steps:
   a. Using the Internet as your tool, make travel arrangements for Dr. Meyer to attend a medical meeting in Montreal, Canada, on June 25-30. She needs to be in Montreal by 4:30 p.m. on June 25 and needs to return home by 6 p.m. on June 30.
   b. Decide on the best flight to meet Dr. Meyer's needs from your site of practice. Record the fare, times of departure and arrival, and any special identification or security requirements.
   c. Make arrangements for Dr. Meyer at a hotel (one of your choosing) for the nights indicated, showing the room fee.
   d. Finally, arrange for land transportation for Dr. Meyer from the airport to the hotel.

2. Travel restrictions and requirements change frequently, particularly for travel outside of the United States. Using the Internet as a resource, locate websites that provide updated information on security, restrictions, and requirements for travelers.

3. Dr. Meyer is scheduled to present a speech on sleep apnea at the June meeting in Montreal. She asks you to consult the Internet and find five links she can use as information resources as she prepares her speech. What did you find?

**Exercise 5**

 **Writing Activity—Maintaining Liability Insurance**

15 minutes

1. Why is liability insurance important in the medical office?

2. What other ways can the medical assistant protect patients from injury in the medical office? List five ways the medical assistant can reduce the chance of accidents.

3. Why is it important for the person responsible for liability insurance to keep a "tickler" file of the dates when premiums are due?

# Telephone Techniques

⚭ **Reading Assignment:** Chapter 5—Interpersonal Skills and Human Behavior
  • The Process of Communication
Chapter 9—Telephone Techniques

**Patients:** Louise Parlet, Wilson Metcalf

**Objectives:**

- Describe how nonverbal and verbal communication are apparent when using the telephone.
- Discuss the need for ethical and legal behavior on the telephone.
- Describe the need for confidentiality when using the telephone in the medical office.

**Overview:**

In this lesson, the legal and ethical issues related to the use of the telephone will be discussed. Issues of confidentiality when using the phone to make arrangements for transfer of a patient to an inpatient facility will also be covered. Proper telephone techniques are important in setting the mood for the entire office. This lesson is designed to provide basic understanding of these techniques.

### Exercise 1

 **CD-ROM Activity—Proper Use of the Telephone in the Medical Office**

 30 minutes

- Sign in to Mountain View Clinic.
- From the patient list, select **Louise Parlet**.

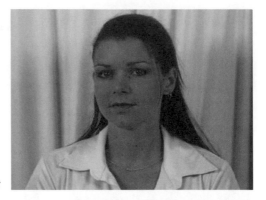

*Louise Parlet*

- On the office map, highlight and click on **Reception** to enter the Reception area.

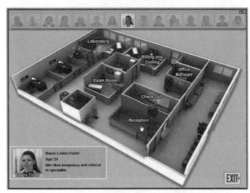

*Click on Reception.*

- Under the Watch heading, select **Patient Check-In** to view the video clip.

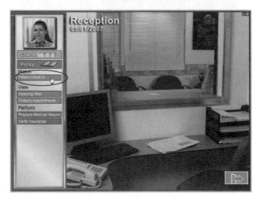

*Click on Patient Check-In*

- At the end of the video, click **Close** to return to the Reception desk.

1. As Kristin answers the phone, how does she identify herself? If this identification a correct procedure? Why or why not?

2. What nonverbal communication does Kristin convey when she answers the phone?

3. Kristin did not close the privacy window while talking on the telephone. Was this a break in confidentiality? Why or why not?

4. When should the privacy window be closed when the medical assistant is on the telephone?

5. Kristin asked Louise Parlet if she could answer the telephone. Was this a proper telephone technique? Give a reason for your answer.

6. Assume that Kristin is engaged in a phone call that involves personal information about the medical condition of a patient. How can she determine whether she is communicating with a person to whom she can legally and ethically release the information?

➤ • Click the exit arrow to go to the Summary Menu.
  • On the Summary Menu, click **Return to Map**.

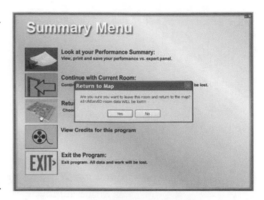

*Click on Return to Map.*

• From the patient list, select Wilson Metcalf.

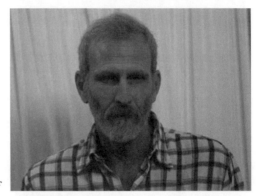

*Wilson Metcalf*

• On the office map, highlight and click on **Check Out**.

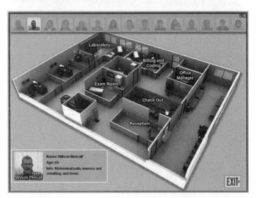

*Click on Check Out.*

• Under the Watch heading, click on **Patient Check-Out** to view the video clip.

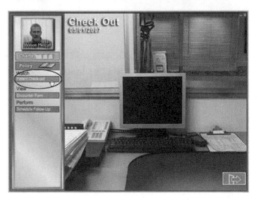

*Click on Patient Check-Out.*

7. How is Mr. Metcalf's confidentiality safeguarded while the medical assistant is on the telephone?

8. How did the medical assistant verify the exact location of the patient transfer so that the orders could be sent as needed?

→ • If you have not already closed the video, click **Close** to return to the Check Out desk.

• At the Check Out desk, click on **Charts** and then on the **Patient Medical Information** tab. Select **7-Release of Information Authorization** from the drop-down menu.

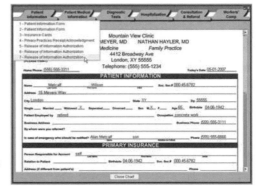

*Click on*
*7-Release of Information Authorization.*

9. Was it permissable for Leah to call Mr. Metcalf's son concerning his transfer to the hospital? Why or why not?

# 3

# Scheduling and Managing Appointments

---

**Reading Assignment:** Chapter 10—Scheduling Appointments

**Patient:** Janet Jones

**Objectives:**

- Discuss the rationale for providing space in a day's appointment schedule for emergency appointments.
- Explain the need for a matrix on the appointment schedule.
- Describe the role of the Policy Manual in appointment scheduling.
- Explain the importance of verbal communication concerning appointment delays.
- Apply the skills of scheduling appointments in person and by telephone.
- Apply the skills of maintaining the appointment book.
- Identify office policies concerning rescheduling appointments.
- Apply the skills of rescheduling appointments.

**Overview:**

In this lesson you will schedule and manage appointments using the policies established for this office. The patient, Janet Jones, is upset because she has not been seen immediately. You will discuss the proper way to deal with such a situation. After today's appointment, Janet Jones will need to come back for a follow-up appointment. You will schedule this appointment for her at the appropriate time.

**Exercise 1**

  **CD-ROM Activity—Using a Specific Daily Appointment Schedule**

20 minutes

- Sign in to Mountain View Clinic
- From the patient list, select Janet Jones.

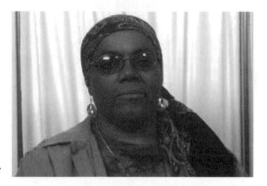

*Janet Jones*

- On the office map, highlight and click on **Reception**.

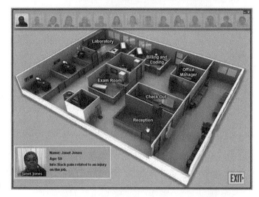

*Click on Reception.*

- At the Reception desk, click **Today's Appointments** (under the View heading) to open the appointment book. Review the scheduled appointments.

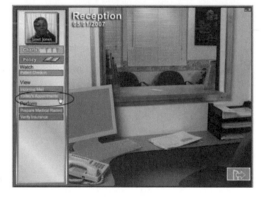

*Click on Today's Appointments.*

- Click **Finish** to close the appointment book and return to the Reception desk.

1. According to the appointment schedule, what time is Janet Jones' appointment?

2. If Janet Jones signed in at 1:30 p.m., would she have been on time for her appointment? Explain your answer.

• Under the Watch heading, click **Patient Check-In** and watch the video.
 • Click **Close** at the end of the video to return to the Reception desk.

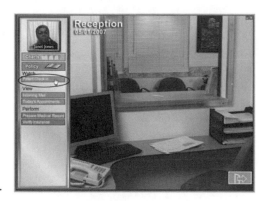

*Click on Patient Check-In.*

3. Janet Jones is upset when she arrives at the counter. How does Kristin handle the patient in a professional way through verbal and nonverbal communication?

4. Assuming that Ms. Jones checked in at 1:30 p.m., what would have been an appropriate statement for the receptionist to make as the patient checked in to prevent her from becoming so upset?

• At the Reception desk, click on **Policy** to open the office Policy Manual.

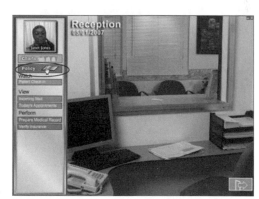

*Click on Policy.*

• Type "appointment scheduling" in the search bar and click once on the magnifying glass.

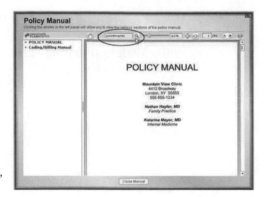

*Search for "appointment scheduling."*

• Read the section of the Policy Manual on scheduling appointments.

5. What is the length of time needed for an appointment during which a history and physical examination must be completed for a new patient?

6. Why is it necessary to set up a matrix before making appointments?

7. What buffer times are available for emergency appointments?

8. According to the office Policy Manual, what would have been appropriate concerning rescheduling this patient's appointment?

9. Why is it important to identify Workers' Compensation appointments at the time of scheduling rather than at the time of the appointment?

→ • Click **Close Manual** to return to the Reception desk.
• Leave **Reception** by clicking the exit arrow at the lower right corner of the screen.

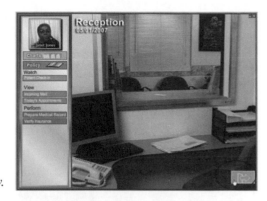

*Click the exit arrow.*

• At the Summary Menu, select **Return to Map** and continue to the next exercise.

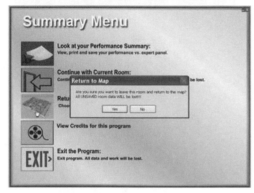

*Click on Return to Map.*

## Exercise 2

 **Writing Activity—Adding Appointments to a Schedule**

 20 minutes

At the end of the day on April 31, a list of patients needing appointments on May 1 was shown to Dr. Hayler and Dr. Meyer. Both physicians stated that because few patients were currently in the hospital, they would be able to see patients in the clinic earlier than usual the next morning. Dr. Hayler and Dr. Meyer will begin seeing patients at 8:15 a.m. The staff has been informed of the early start.

1. a. Insert the following appointments for Dr. Hayler into the morning schedule on the next page.

   (1) Robert Leuker is a patient who has not been to the clinic in 5 years and wants to be seen for a lump in his arm. He has a past history of cancer and needs to be seen ASAP. He should be seen first in the morning so that he can be referred as necessary. He is insured through BlueCross/BlueShield (BC/BS).

   (2) Lindsey Repp needs a follow-up appointment for an earache and recurrent fever. She is insured through Central Health HMO and can be double-booked at the end of the appointment for Louise Parlet.

   (3) John Price, who needs a follow-up appointment for his blood pressure, has Medicare. His blood pressure was low when he took it yesterday, and he feels dizzy. He simply wants Dr. Hayler to reevaluate his medication. He can be seen just before lunch.

| 5/1/20XX | Dr. Hayler | | | Dr. Meyer | |
|---|---|---|---|---|---|
| Time | Patient Name | Insurance | | Patient Name | Insurance |
| 8:00 AM | (Hospital rounds)<br>Joe Smitty - Chem 12, CBC<br>Marsha Brady - Fasting BS | | | (Hospital Rounds) | |
| 8:15 AM | (Hospital rounds) | | | (Hospital Rounds)<br><br>Joanne Crosby, PT, PTT | |
| 8:30 AM | Louise Parlet, Est. Pt<br>New Pregnancy/Pelvic<br>(555) 555-3214 | Teachers | | Rhea Davison, Est. Pt.<br>Elevated BS, abdominal<br>distention, pelvic (555) 555-5656 | None |
| 8:45 AM | | | | | |
| 9:00 AM | | | | | |
| 9:15 AM | | | | | |
| 9:30 AM | | | | Hu Huang, Est. Pt.<br>Severe cough, fever<br>(555) 555-1454 | Medicare |
| 9:45 AM | Jade Wong, NP<br>7 mos well child checkup/<br>immunization (555) 555-3345 | Central Health<br><br>HMO | | | |
| 10:00 AM | | | | ~~Chris O'Neill back pain~~<br>(pt cancelled - resched 5/7)<br>Jesus Santo, Walk-in Leg pain, SOB | None |
| 10:15 AM | | | | | |
| 10:30 AM | | | | Jean Deere, Est. Pt.<br>Memory loss, ear pain<br>(555) 555-6361 | Medicare |
| 10:45 AM | Tristan Tsosie, Est. Pt.<br>Suture Removal<br>(555) 555-1515 | Blue Cross/<br>Blue Shield | | | |
| 11:00 AM | | | | | |
| 11:15 AM | | | | Wilson Metcalf, Est. Pt.<br>N/V, abdominal pain, difficulty<br>urinating - (555) 555-3311 | Medicare |
| 11:30 AM | LUNCH | | | | |
| 11:45 AM | | | | | |
| 12:00 PM | | | | | |
| 12:15 PM | Renee Anderson, NP<br>Annual GYN Exam<br>(555) 555-3331 | Blue Cross/<br>Blue Shield | | | |

b. After completing Dr. Hayler's appointments, add the following appointments for Dr. Meyer in the morning, using the same schedule on the previous page.

(1) Catherine Lake needs a follow-up appointment for pyelonephritis. She forgot to make her follow-up appointment when she was last seen. Ms. Lake is going out of town for 2 weeks and needs to see Dr. Meyer before leaving. Her insurance coverage is through BC/BS. Dr. Meyer will see her at the earliest appointment time.

(2) Lucille Meryl needs to be seen for a follow-up to a thyroid test. Dr. Meyer wants to see her as a double-booking at the end of the appointment for Rhea Davison. Her insurance is through Drake.

(3) An established patient, Simon Reed, calls at 11:30 a.m. to tell you that he has some chest pain, and even though he has an appointment for tomorrow, he does not think he should wait. When you discuss this with Dr. Meyer, she tells you to book him ASAP. Mr. Reed, who has BC/BS insurance, tells you that it will take him about 20 minutes to get to the office.

2. You must now call John Price to inform him that Dr. Hayler will see him just before lunch. Write the information below that Mr. Price will need to be told. Why did Dr. Hayler need to be contacted before making the appointment for Mr. Price?

3. You must also call Lucille Meryl to inform her that Dr. Meyer wants to see her about her test results. What information do you need to provide, and how would you answer her when she questions why she needs to be seen so quickly?

**Exercise 3**

 **CD-ROM Activity—Preparing an Appointment Schedule**

 30 minutes

- In this exercise we will continue with Janet Jones' visit. If you are already at the office map, click on **Check Out** to go to the Check Out desk. (*Note:* If you have exited the program, sign in again to Mountain View Clinic, select Janet Jones, and go to the Check Out desk.)

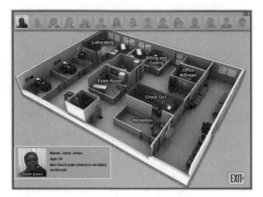

*Click on Check Out.*

- At the Check Out desk, click **Encounter Form** under the View heading.

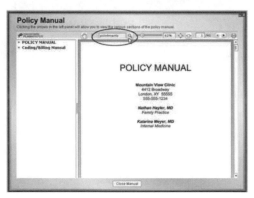

*Click on Encounter Form.*

1. What is the date that Janet Jones should return to the clinic for a follow-up appointment?

2. How much time should be allotted to the follow-up appointment for Ms. Jones?

3. Complete the following activities using the appointment sheets on the next two pages.

    (1)  Set up the appointment sheet for the date that Janet Jones is to return for her follow-up visit.

    (2)  Using the information in the Policy Manual, set up the matrix for that day. (*Note:* If you need to review this, return to the Policy Manual, type "hours of operation" in the search bar, and click once on the magnifying glass.)

    (3)  Before entering an appointment for Janet Jones, add an appointment at 11:00 a.m. for Kay Soto (an established patient) with Dr. Meyer. Ms. Soto has been prescribed a weight loss program and is coming in for a weight check. Her insurance is through Metro HMO.

Continue adding appointments to the schedule using the list provided at the top of page 12.

## Appointment Book, Page 1

| /__/20XX | Dr. Hayler | | Dr. Meyer | |
|---|---|---|---|---|
| Time | Patient Name | Insurance | Patient Name | Insurance |
| 8:00 AM | | | | |
| 8:15 AM | | | | |
| 8:30 AM | | | | |
| 8:45 AM | | | | |
| 9:00 AM | | | | |
| 9:15 AM | | | | |
| 9:30 AM | | | | |
| 9:45 AM | | | | |
| 10:00 AM | | | | |
| 10:15 AM | | | | |
| 10:30 AM | | | | |
| 10:45 AM | | | | |
| 11:00 AM | | | | |
| 11:15 AM | | | | |
| 11:30 AM | | | | |
| 11:45 AM | | | | |
| 12:00 PM | | | | |
| 12:15 PM | | | | |

4.

## Appointment Book, Page 2

| /   /20XX | Dr. Hayler | | Dr. Meyer | |
|---|---|---|---|---|
| Time | Patient Name | Insurance | Patient Name | Insurance |
| 12:30 PM | | | | |
| 12:45 PM | | | | |
| 1:00 PM | | | | |
| 1:15 PM | | | | |
| 1:30 PM | | | | |
| 1:45 PM | | | | |
| 2:00 PM | | | | |
| 2:15 PM | | | | |
| 2:30 PM | | | | |
| 2:45 PM | | | | |
| 3:00 PM | | | | |
| 3:15 PM | | | | |
| 3:30 PM | | | | |
| 3:45 PM | | | | |
| 4:00 PM | | | | |
| 4:15 PM | | | | |
| 4:30 PM | | | | |
| 4:45 PM | | | | |
| 5:00 PM | | | | |

Continue your scheduling by adding the following appointments to the forms on the previous two pages.

(4) George Smith, age 15, is to be seen by Dr. Hayler for a football injury the night before. He has State Agricultural Insurance and is an existing patient. George needs to be seen as early as possible so that he can go to school.

(5) Callie Agree, a new patient, is to be seen for a possible sinus infection. She has Medicare and will be accompanied by her daughter. The daughter prefers to see Dr. Meyer in the midmorning so that her mother will have time to dress.

(6) Sophie Coats, age 6 months, is an established patient who will be seen by Dr. Hayler for a well-baby visit. She is due to have immunizations at this visit. Her mother prefers to have an appointment as early in the morning as possible. Sophie is covered by her father's insurance with Banker's Health.

(7) Mamie Mack, age 18, is an established patient who needs a physical for college. She prefers to be seen by Dr. Hayler. Either late morning or early afternoon is better for her since she is still in school. She is covered through George Allen Insurance at her mother's place of employment.

(8) Kay Soto calls to cancel her appointment for the day because she has to leave town to take care of her ill mother. She does not want to reschedule at this time.

(9) Make the appointment for Janet Jones for her follow-up visit.

(10) Dr. Hayler will need to leave at 11:15 for a dental appointment but will be back in the afternoon. Mark this on the appointment sheet.

(11) Dr. Meyer is scheduled to be off the afternoon of this day. Mark this on the appointment sheet.

5. What are the necessary procedures for canceling Kay Soto's appointment?
   a. Erase the canceled appointment and tell Ms. Soto that there will be a charge because she did not give 24 hours' notice.
   b. Cross out the appointment (using the office-preferred writing implement) and record the cancellation in the patient medical record.
   c. Report the cancellation to Dr. Meyer.
   d. Tell Kay Soto that she must reschedule this appointment today for continued medical care.

# Scheduling Admissions and Procedures

/OͲ **Reading Assignment:** Chapter 10—Scheduling Appointments
- Scheduling Other Types of Appointments

Chapter 14—Documentation and Medical Records Management
- Releasing Medical Record Information

**Patients:** Wilson Metcalf, Shaunti Begay

**Objectives:**

- Recognize the information needed when transferring a patient to a hospital from a medical office.
- Explain the importance of confidentiality when admitting a patient to the hospital.
- Discuss why it is important for patients to understand the need for proper preparation for outpatient admissions and testing.
- Explain the importance of giving patients accurate directions to outpatient facilities.
- Identify the information needed for outpatient admissions and testing.
- Explain why it is important to arrange outpatient appointments at a time convenient for the patient.
- Discuss ethical boundaries that must be recognized during hospital admissions and referrals.

**Overview:**

In this lesson you will make the necessary arrangements for moving Wilson Metcalf from the office to the hospital. You will ensure that his family has been notified of the move. With Shaunti Begay, you will make arrangements for outpatient testing and schedule an office appointment for providing her test results. This patient will also need to see a specialist, so any questions concerning the insurance for these appointments will need to be answered.

### Exercise 1

  **CD-ROM Activity—Scheduling Inpatient Admissions and Procedures**

30 minutes

- Sign in to Mountain View Clinic.
- From the patient list, select **Wilson Metcalf**.

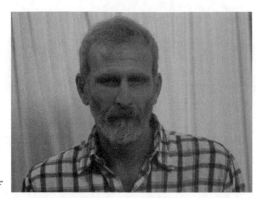

*Wilson Metcalf*

- On the office map, highlight and click on **Check Out**.

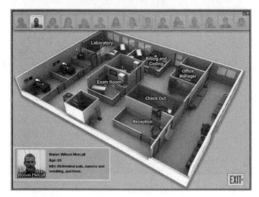

*Click on Check Out.*

- Click on **Policy** to open the office Policy Manual.
- Type "job description" in the search bar and click once on the magnifying glass.
- Read the section of the Policy Manual concerning the job descriptions for the medical assistants.

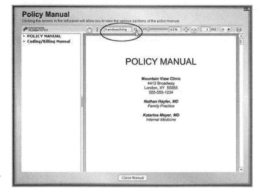

*Search for "job description."*

1. According to office policy, which medical assistant has the primary duty of making the arrangements for inpatient admissions and for making referrals to other physicians?

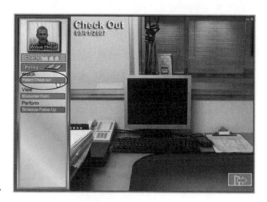

- Click **Close Manual** to return to the Check Out desk.
- Under the Watch heading, select **Patient Check-Out** to view the video. At the end of the video, click **Close**.

*Select Patient Check-Out.*

2. Which documents are being copied and sent to the hospital with Mr. Metcalf?

_____ Medicare card

_____ Private insurance card

_____ Authorization form

_____ Office registration

_____ Physician's orders

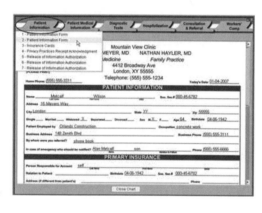

- Click on **Charts** to open Wilson Metcalf's medical record.
- Next, click on the **Patient Information** tab.
- From the drop-down menu, select and read the **Patient Information Form** and the **Authorization Form** (both dated 5-1-2007).

*Click on the Patient Information tab.*

- Click **Close Chart** when you have finished reviewing the documents.

3. Why would it be appropriate to send the office registration and authorization form to the hospital for Wilson Metcalf's admission?

4. Who may receive information concerning Mr. Metcalf's medical condition? Can the entire medical record be released?

5. Did Leah act within the ethical and legal boundaries to release the information she gave to the hospital for Mr. Metcalf? Explain your answer.

6. Why is it important that the window to the waiting room be closed while Leah is making arrangements for Mr. Metcalf to be transferred to the hospital?

7. In March, Mr. Metcalf had a upper GI series with a small bowel follow-up at Braeburn Medical Center. Describe the necessary steps for the medical assistant to make the appointment for this procedure.

→ • Under the Perform heading, click on **Schedule Follow-Up**.

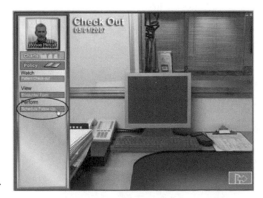

*Click on Schedule Follow-Up.*

- Select the actions that you feel are needed for Mr. Metcalf's follow-up. Click **Finish** when you are satisfied with your answers.
- Click on the exit arrow at the bottom of screen.
- From the Summary Menu, click on **Look at Your Performance Summary** to compare your answers with those of the experts.

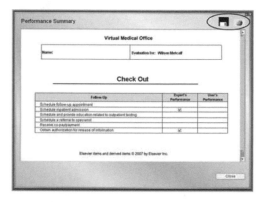

*Select Look at Your Performance Summary.*

- You may save and/or print your Performance Summary by clicking on the icons in the upper right corner of the screen.

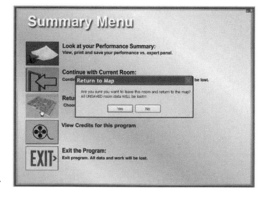

*Print and/or save your report.*

- Click **Close**.
- From the Summary Menu, select **Return to Map**. (*Remember:* If you did not save your Performance Summary, all data will be lost when you return to the map.)

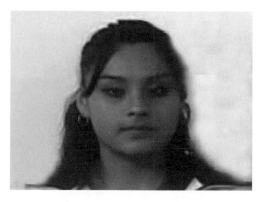

*Click on Return to Map.*

## Exercise 2

###  CD-ROM Activity—Scheduling Outpatient Admissions and Procedures

 This exercise will take approximately 20 minutes to complete.

- From the patient list, select **Shaunti Begay**. (*Note:* If you have exited the program, sign in again to Mountain View Clinic and select Shaunti Begay from the patient list.)

*Shaunti Begay*

- Highlight and click on **Check Out** on the office map.

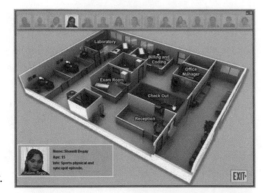

*Click on Check Out.*

- Select **Charts** to open Shaunti Begay's medical record.

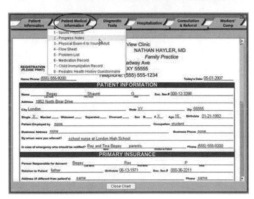

*Click on Charts.*

- Under the **Patient Medical Information** tab, select **2-Progress Notes** to read the documentation on the current visit.

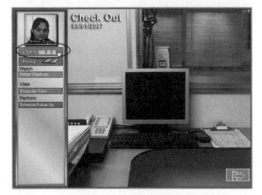

*Select 2-Progress Notes.*

1. What appointments does the check-out medical assistant need to make?

- Click **Close Chart**.
- Under the Watch heading, select **Patient Check-Out** to view the video.

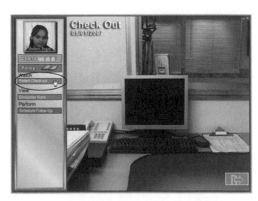

*Click on Patient Check-Out.*

• When you have finished watching the video, click **Close**.

2. Did Leah make sure the referral for outpatient admission and procedures was scheduled at a time convenient for the patient and her family?

3. Why is it important to check that referrals and appointments to specialists are made at a time that is convenient for the patient?

4. Shaunti's father, Mr. Begay, is concerned with the financial aspects of the visit since his insurance is not a provider for this medical office. Leah provided the information about his insurance carrier and the referral. However, she did not provide information that was needed to assist Shaunti in the referral. Can you name two items that were not discussed with or given to Mr. Begay?

5. Mr. Begay was concerned about the amount of the bill for Shaunti. Do you think that Leah was professional in her handling of verbal and nonverbal communication in this interaction? In what way, if any, would you have changed what was said or done? Did Leah act in an ethical manner?

• Under the Perform heading, click on **Schedule Follow-Up**.

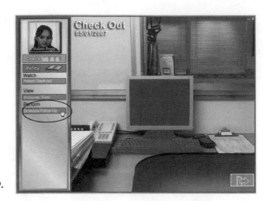

*Click on Schedule Follow-Up.*

• Complete the checklist and click **Finish**.
• Click on exit arrow at bottom of screen to leave the area.
• On the Summary Menu, select **Look at Your Performance Summary** to compare your answers with those of the experts.

# Maintaining a Proper Inventory

**Reading Assignment:** Chapter 12—The Office Environment and Daily Operations
- Supplies and Equipment in the Physician's Office

Chapter 14—Documentation and Medical Records Management
- Supplies

**Patients:** None

**Objectives:**

- Describe the steps necessary for replenishing supplies.
- Discuss how having too many or too few supplies can affect the efficiency of the office.
- Decide which items to reorder and the amount to reorder.
- Explain the necessity of checking equipment for maintenance on a regular basis.
- Discuss the role of the medical assistant in suggesting new equipment for the medical office.
- Describe the proper disposal of controlled substances that are found to be out of date.

**Overview:**

Ensuring the availability of supplies and equipment when needed is essential to the efficiency of the medical office practice. The proper inventory of supplies and equipment helps to ensure their availability. In some cases, it is more efficient to order supplies in larger quantities. The medical assistant also has the responsibility of making sure that the equipment ordered is the most currently used in the field. Finally, when medications are found to be out of date, proper disposal is necessary. This lesson will focus on supplies and equipment and their importance to office efficiency.

### Exercise 1

 **CD-ROM Activity—Deciding When to Replenish Supplies**

 30 minutes

• Sign in to Mountain View Clinic.

• On the office map, highlight and click on **Office Manager** to enter the manager's office. (*Note:* You do not need to select a patient for this exercise.)

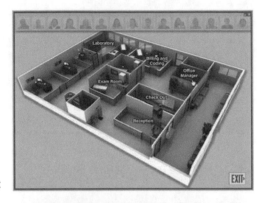

*Click on Office Manger.*

• Click on **Supply Inventory** to view the inventory records.

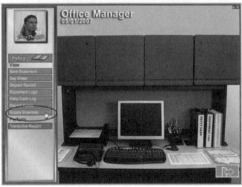

*Click on Supply Inventory.*

• To view the record for each item in inventory, click on the corresponding tab headings.

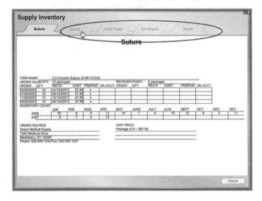

*Click on tab headings to view each item.*

1. What is the reorder point for sutures?

2. Looking at the record from 2006, how many packages of sutures were previously used in May?

3. Should sutures be reordered? If so, why and how many? If not, why not?

➜ • Click on the tab heading for **Gauze** to view the inventory record.

4. What is the reorder point for gauze?

5. Looking at the record from 2006, how many bags of gauze were previously used in May?

6. The inventory for gauze is recorded as bags, but gauze can also be ordered by the case. How many bags are in one case?

7. What is the unit price? Does this represent the price per bag or the price per case?

8. What is the discount offered for ordering four or more cases of gauze?

9. After looking at the inventory supply sheet for gauze, should gauze be reordered? If so, why and how much? If not, why not? If you reorder, what will be the net amount of the purchase?

➡ • Click on the tab heading for **EKG Paper** to view the inventory record.

10. When was the last order placed for EKG paper? How much was ordered?

11. When was this order received?

12. What is the reorder point for EKG paper?

13. How many packs of EKG paper are currently in inventory?

14. Should EKG paper be reordered now? If so, why? If not, why not? If you reorder, what quantity should be reordered?

15. The order for EKG paper is prepaid. What are some possible reasons for setting up a prepaid order for this item?

➤ • Click on the tab heading for **Envelopes** to view the inventory record.

16. How often does the office normally order envelopes?

17. On January 15, 2007, the office received an order of four boxes of envelopes. Assuming only one of the boxes from this order was used in January and another two boxes were used in February, how many boxes of envelopes were in inventory on March 1, 2007?

18. On February 28, 2007, the office ordered four more boxes of envelopes. When did this order arrive?

19. Why is there so much time between when the order is placed and when the order is received?

20. From what you see on the inventory form, do the envelopes need to be reordered? How could the office lower the price of the envelopes? Do you see a problem with the reorder point, and does this need to be changed? If the envelopes should be reordered in bulk, what would be the price?

➤ • Click on the tab heading for **Paper** to view the inventory record for copier paper.

21. After examining the inventory supply card for copier paper, what amount of paper do you think should be ordered to meet the order quantity? How much would the paper cost?

22. For the purpose of this exercise, we will assume all supplies can be ordered through the same vendor. Complete the purchase order below to order the necessary items you have identified in this exercise. Include a 6% sales tax and $12.00 for shipping.

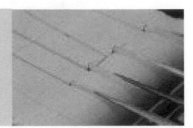

# All Purpose Medical Supply

## Purchase Order

Bill To:
Mountain View Clinic
4412 Broadway
London, XY 55555

Ship To:
Mountain View Clinic
4412 Broadway
London, XY 55555

Order #: 105699
Date:

Delivery Required By:

| Sales Contact | Terms | Tax ID |
|---|---|---|
|  |  |  |

| Item | Quantity | Description | Unit Price | Disc % | Total |
|---|---|---|---|---|---|
|  |  |  |  |  |  |
|  |  |  |  |  |  |
|  |  |  |  |  |  |
|  |  |  |  |  |  |
|  |  |  |  |  |  |
|  |  |  |  |  |  |
|  |  |  |  |  |  |
|  |  |  |  |  |  |
|  |  |  |  |  |  |
|  |  |  |  |  |  |
|  |  |  |  |  |  |
|  |  |  |  |  |  |

| | |
|---|---|
| Shipping |  |
| Subtotal |  |
| Tax % |  |
| Balance Due |  |

999 Vendor Road, Industrial Park, XY 55555
Phone: (123) 456 7890 Fax: (123) 456 7899 CSR@allpurpose.com

23. How should the ordered supplies be handled when they arrive at the office?

24.

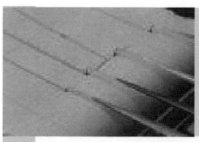

# All Purpose Medical Supply

## INVOICE # 2297

DATE:
Customer Name: Mountain View Clinic

| BILL TO: | SHIP TO: |
|---|---|
| COMPANY NAME:<br>Mountain View Clinic | COMPANY NAME:<br>Mountain View Clnic |
| COMPANY ADDRESS:<br>4412 Broadway<br>London, XY 55555 | COMPANY ADDRESS:<br>4412 Broadway<br>London, XY 55555 |

| Order # | Sales Contact | Terms | Tax ID |
|---|---|---|---|
| 105699 | | | |

| Item | Quantity | Description | Unit Price | Disc % | Total |
|---|---|---|---|---|---|
| NE562 | 4 cases | 4x4 Stretch Gauze | $23.58/case | 10% | $103.66 |
| Ltr-009 | 10 boxes | Custom printed window envelopes | $23.10/box | 20% | $277.20 |
| CPO-117 | 3 cases | Copier Paper | $71.27/3 cases | | $71.27 |
| | | | | | |
| | | | | | |
| | | | | | |
| | | | | | |
| | | | | | |
| | | | | | |
| | | | | | |
| | | | | | |
| | | | | | |

| | |
|---|---|
| Shipping | 12.00 |
| Subtotal | $464.13 |
| Tax % | $27.84 |
| Balance Due | $491.97 |

999 Vendor Road, Industrial Park, XY 55555
Phone: (123) 456 7890 Fax: (123) 456 7899 CSR@allpurpose.com

Using the information on the invoice above, complete the check on the next page to pay for the the delivered supplies.

173980

DATE:_____

TO: _____

FOR: _____

ACCOUNT NO. _____

| AMOUNT PAID | $ |

MOUNTAIN VIEW CLINIC
4412 Broadway
London, XY 55555

173980

94-72/1224

Date: _____

Pay to the order of: _____

_____ Dollars   $ _____

Clarion National Bank
Member FDIC
90 Grape Vine Road
London, XY 55555-0001

Authorized Signature

‖ 005509 ‖ 446782011 ‖ 678800470

## Exercise 2

### Writing Activity—Properly Disposing Medications

10 minutes

1. While checking supplies, Cathy noticed that some of the nonscheduled medications are out of date. These medications are oral tablets and capsules. What means of disposal is correct for these medications?

2. Cathy also found some Schedule II medications that are out of date. What is the correct procedure for disposal of these medications?

## Exercise 3

### Writing Activity—Maintaining Administrative Equipment

10 minutes

1. When filling the copier with paper, Cathy notices that it is time for regular maintenance of the machine and the representative has not been to the office. What should be Cathy's next step?

2. The toner cartridges are low, and Cathy sees a need for replenishing these. What should she do?

## Exercise 4

### Writing Activity—Suggestions for Equipment and Supplies

10 minutes

Ameeta has observed that not all patients with diabetes are using the same glucose meters at home. The physicians are asking that quality control be checked with patients more often. However, if the office does not have the same glucometers and supplies that some of the patients use at home, it is difficult to provide accurate patient teaching.

1. What steps should Ameeta take to ensure that patient teaching is accurate and helpful to each patient?

2. Leah, as an administrative assistant, has found that the phone line for the fax machine is often busy when a fax needs to be received. Often the person attempting to send the fax has called to complain of the difficulty of getting important information to the physicians. What steps should Leah take to show the need for another fax line for the hospital?

# Written Communications

---

⌐○⌐○ **Reading Assignment:** Chapter 13—Written Communication and Document Processing

**Patient:** Wilson Metcalf

**Objectives:**

- Prepare letters in response to the mail received.
- Use correct grammar, spelling, and formatting techniques in letter writing.
- Use correct medical terminology as appropriate.
- Answer mail appropriately and promptly.
- Transcribe medical records.

**Overview:**

In this lesson you will be asked to respond to incoming mail that includes an NSF check and a letter from a collection agency. The maintenance of liability insurance must be verified with a letter to be faxed to the insurance company. Also in this lesson, you will transcribe a medical record.

## Exercise 1

 **CD-ROM Activity—Composing a Letter for an NSF Check**

 30 minutes

- Sign into Mountain View Clinic.
- From the patient list, select **Wilson Metcalf**.

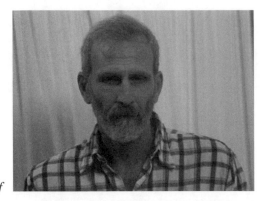

*Wilson Metcalf*

- On the office map, highlight and click on **Reception** to enter the Reception area.

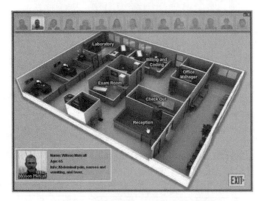

*Click on Reception.*

- Under the View heading, select **Incoming Mail** to view the mail received by the clinic.

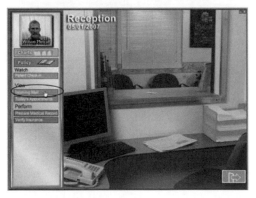

*Click on Incoming Mail.*

- From the list of mail at the top of the screen, click on **7** to view that piece of mail.

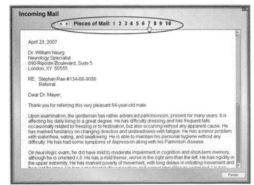

*Click on 7.*

• Compose a letter for the NSF check using the document in the transcription wizard in the office manager. Be sure to include the service charge.

• Leave the Incoming Mail window open as you complete the remaining exercises.

1. Below, write your letter to the patient about the NSF check, using an acceptable format. Be sure your message conveys the need to handle this matter within a certain number of days. Also include that no further checks will be accepted for this patient's medical care at Mountain View Clinic. This should be prepared for a signature by the office manager.

**Mountain View Clinic**

4412 Broadway / London, XY 55555 / Phone: (555) 555-1234 / Fax (555) 555-1239

*Nathan Hayler, MD - Family Practice / Katarina Meyer, MD - Internal Medicine*

### Exercise 2

### CD-ROM Activity—Composing a Letter in Response to an Inaccurate Accounts Payable

15 minutes

- From the list of mail at the top of the screen, click on **10** to read the letter from Summer Oxygen Company.
- Click **Finish** to return to the Reception Desk.

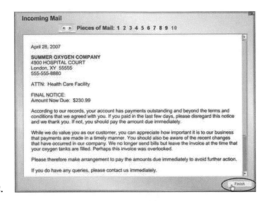

*Click on Finish.*

- Click the exit arrow to leave the Reception area.
- On the Summary Menu, click **Return to Map**.

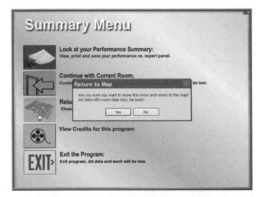

*Click Return to Map.*

- On the office map, highlight and click on **Office Manager** to enter the manager's office.

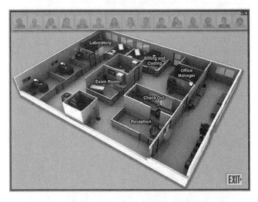

*Click on Office Manager.*

- Under the View heading, click on **Bank Statement** to view the most recent statement from the bank.

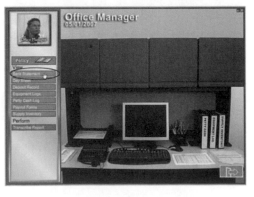

*Click on Bank Statement.*

• Select the **Check Ledger** tab to review the most recent checks written by Mountain View Clinic.

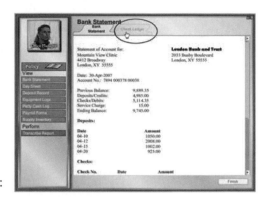

*Click on Check Ledger.*

1. There was a payment made to Summer Oxygen Company for $230.99.

   a. According to the check ledger, what was the date the payment was made?

   b. What was the check number?

 • Click on the **Bank Statement** tab to review the account activity for April, 2007.

   2. Did check #1230 for $230.99 clear the account, according to the bank statement?

 • Compose a letter to the oxygen supply company in response to the claim that the invoice has not been paid. Be sure to include in the correspondence that a copy of the canceled check is enclosed with the letter.

   • Click **Finish** to return to the manager's office.

3. Below, write your letter to the oxygen company using an acceptable format. Be sure your message includes all information needed to clear the accounts payable. This should be prepared for signature by the office manager.

**Mountain View Clinic**

4412 Broadway / London, XY 55555 / Phone: (555) 555-1234 / Fax: (555) 555-1239

*Nathan Hayler, MD - Family Practice / Katarina Meyer, MD - Internal Medicine*

## Exercise 3

 **CD-ROM Activity—Medical Transcription**

 30 minutes

- In the manager's office, click on **Transcribe Report** to access the dictated report.

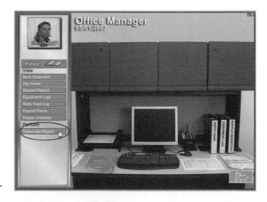

*Click on Transcribe Report.*

- Review the instructions on how to operate the player and transcribe the discharge report as dictated, using the dates on the recording.
- Be sure that you use the correct format, grammar, style, and medical terminology.
- Click **Print** for a hard copy of your transcription. Click **Finish** to close the player.

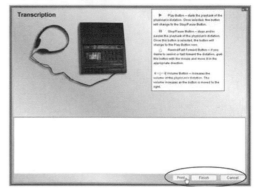

*Click Finish to close the player.*

# Organizing a Patient's Medical Record

**Reading Assignment:** Chapter 14—Documentation and Medical Records Management
- Organization of the Medical Record
- Contents of the Complete Case History
- Making Additions to the Patient Record
- Keeping Records Current

**Patients:** Renee Anderson, Tristan Tsosie

## Objectives:

- Discuss why proper organization of the medical record is essential.
- Identify and describe the forms found in a medical record.
- Apply principles of medical record organization to preparing a new patient's medical record.
- Select the forms that need to be added to the medical record for an established patient.
- Describe the appropriate care of a damaged medical record.
- Determine the appropriate division of medical records when a new record must be established.

## Overview:

In this lesson we will explore the importance of preparing a patient's medical record correctly. Because the medical record is a legal document that shows the chronological care of the patient, this document must be correctly organized to ensure that information can be located as needed. Incorrectly organized charts not only cause frustration, but also decrease the efficiency of the medical practice. In this lesson you will organize a medical record for a new patient. For an established patient, you will ensure that information received from other sources has been properly organized and that the information is readily available when the patient arrives for an appointment.

### Exercise 1

 **CD-ROM Activity—Organizing a Medical Record for a New Patient**

 30 minutes

- Sign in to Mountain View Clinic.
- From the patient list, select **Renee Anderson**.

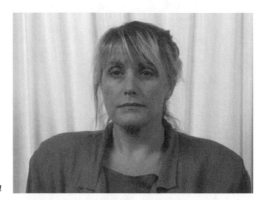

*Renee Anderson*

- Highlight and click on **Reception** on the office map.

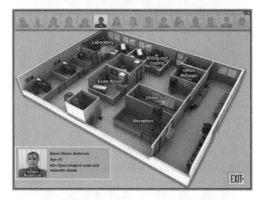

*Click on Reception.*

- Click on **Policy** to open the Policy Manual. In the search bar, type "medical record" and click on the magnifying glass to search.

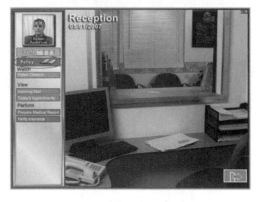

*Click on Policy.*
*Then search for "medical record."*

- Scroll up and down to read the duties assigned to the various types of medical assistants in the office.

1. At Mountain View Clinic, the Policy Manual states that the _____ medical assistant is responsible for preparing and organizing the medical record.

2. Why is it important for the administrative medical assistant to provide the necessary forms in a medical record for a new patient?

→ • When you have finished reading the relevant policy, click on **Close Manual** to return to the Reception desk.

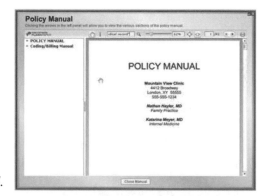

*Click on Close Manual.*

• At the Reception desk, click on **Prepare Medical Record** (under the Perform heading) to begin assembling a chart for Ms. Anderson's visit.

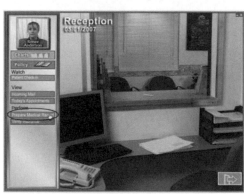

*Click on Prepare Medical Record.*

• Next to Assemble Medical Record, click on **Perform** to begin selecting the forms necessary for Ms. Anderson's visit.

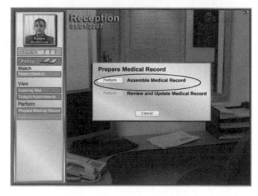

*Click on Perform
(next to Assemble Medical Record).*

• The Patient Information tab is automatically chosen as the starting point when you access the Assemble Medical Record screen. Under Forms Available, choose the forms that should be filed under the Patient Information tab. Click **Add** to complete your selections. (*Note:* To select multiple consecutive forms, hold down the Shift key while making your selections. To make multiple nonconsecutive selections, hold down the Control [Ctrl] key as you click on your choices.)

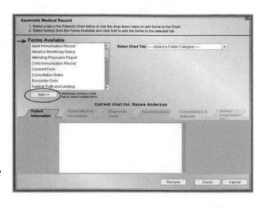

*Make selections from Forms Available and click Add.*

• When you have completed the Patient Information section, continue adding forms to the appropriate tabs in Renee Anderson's medical record. To select a new tab, either click on the tab on the medical record itself or use the drop-down menu to the right of Select Chart Tab.

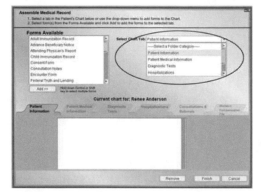

*Select a chart tab to assemble.*

• If you change you mind about a form you have added to a tab, click to highlight the name of the form and then click on **Remove** at the bottom of the screen.

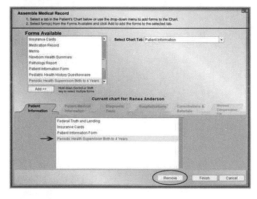

*Click Remove to delete a form.*

• When you are satisfied that you have selected all the necessary forms and put them in the correct tab sections, click **Finish** to close the medical record.

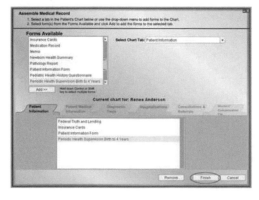

*Click Finish.*

• Now click on the exit arrow at the bottom of screen to leave the Reception area.

• On the Summary Menu, click on **Look at Your Performance Summary** to compare your answers against those of the experts. How did you do?

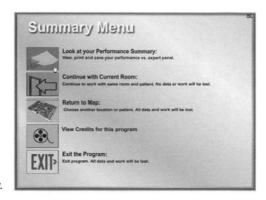

*Click on Look at Your Performance Summary.*

• The icons for saving and printing the Performance Summary are located at the top right corner of the screen.

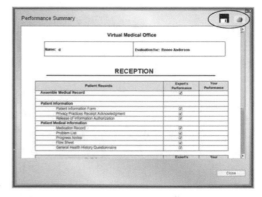

*Save and/or print your summary.*

• Click **Close**.

• Click **Return to Map**. (*Note:* If you did not save your Performance Summary, all data will be lost when you return to the map.)

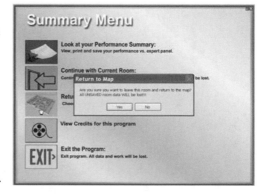

*Click on Return to Map.*

3. The form that contains the patient's demographic information is the

   _____.

4. The form in the medical record that contains subjective information about the patient's

   illnesses in the past is the _____.

5. The legal document that must be signed to allow information to be used to file insurance is

   the _____.

6. The form that allows the physician to record findings in the medical record is the

   _____.

**Exercise 2**

**CD-ROM Activity—Adding to the Medical Record of an Established Patient**

20 minutes

• From the patient list, click on **Tristan Tsosie**. (*Note:* If you have exited the program, sign in again to Mountain View Clinic and select Trsitan Tsosie from the patient list.)

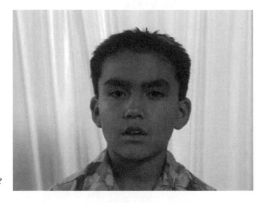

*Tristan Tsosie*

• On the office map, click on **Reception**.
• At the Reception desk, click on **Charts**.
• Click on the **Hospitalization** tab. From the drop-down menu, select **1-ED Record**.

*Click on Hospitalization; then click on 1-ED Record.*

• Read the ED Record to decide what other forms should be available for the physician for this office visit and to determine whether Tristan is following the orders of the physician who saw him in the Emergency Department.
• Click on **Close Chart** to return to the Reception area.
• Under the Perform heading, select **Prepare Medical Record**.
• Click on the **Perform** button next to Review and Update Medical Records.

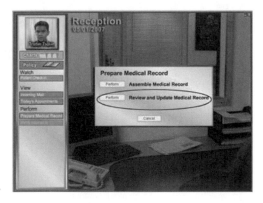

*Review and Update Medical Records.*

• Check the forms in each chart tab to be sure that the needed information for this visit is located under the correct tab and will be available when the physician needs it. Add any forms that you think are needed for this visit. If you think it is necessary, you may also remove or move any forms within the chart. (*Note:* If you need help with these steps, see the detailed instructions in Exercise 1 of this lesson.)

• Click **Finish** when you are done.

1. Was Tristan's follow-up appointment made at the appropriate time as directed by the physician in the Emergency Department?

2. What report(s), other than the ED Record, should have been added to the medical record for it to be complete for the physician?

3. When adding a form to the medical record, the medical assistant should:
   a. be sure the physician has seen the report before filing it.
   b. place the forms in the medical record in chronological order, with the earliest record on top.
   c. always be sure the date of arrival has been stamped on the form.
   d. wait to file the form just before the patient's arrival for an appointment.
   e. do both a and d.

4. When the medical assistant files materials in the medical record of an established patient, the materials should be filed in what order?

5. When accessing Tristan's medical record on arrival, you notice that the forms from the hospital have been torn during transmittal. What steps do you need to take to maintain the record from further damage?

6. If a patient's folder is old, torn, or simply worn, what should the medical assistant do?

7. If a chart is overcrowded and a second chart needs to be established, how far back should the records go that are moved to the new chart? How should the record be marked to show that more than one medical record is available?

# Filing Medical Records

∅⊘ **Reading Assignment:** Chapter 14—Documentation and Medical Records Management
  - Filing Procedures
  - Filing Methods
  - Organization of Files

**Patients:** All

**Objectives:**

- Alphabetize patient names for efficiency in filing medical records.
- List the necessary steps needed to prepare a medical record for filing.
- Describe the use of outguides, colored file folders, color-coded name labels, and aging labels.
- Incorporate correct labeling to provide ease of filing.
- Describe the differences in alphabetic and numeric filing.
- Discuss the need to purge older medical records.
- Discuss means for finding displaced medical records.
- Discuss the importance of using correct filing techniques for time management.

**Overview:**

Proper filing of medical records is essential in providing continuity of care for patients. Lost records prevent the physician from knowing what medical care has been provided in the past and may even be the cause of a malpractice claim. Many offices use visual aids for keeping medical records properly filed, such as color-coded name labels and outguides. Aging labels may be used to assist with purging older medical records.

### Exercise 1

 **CD-ROM Activity—Preparing Patient Medical Records for Filing**

 50 minutes

- Sign in to Mountain View Clinic.
- One at a time, select each patient from the patient list (moving from left to right) and record his or her name in the table in question 1 below.

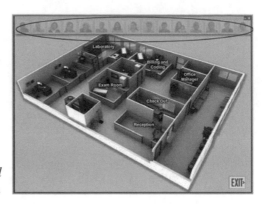

*Select each patient and record his or her name in the table below.*

1. Record the names of the Mountain View Clinic patients in the first and third columns of the table below. Fill in all of column 1 first; then continue at the top of column 3.

| Patient Name | First Date of Service; Last Date of Service | Patient Name | First Date of Service; Last Date of Service |
|---|---|---|---|
| | | | |
| | | | |
| | | | |
| | | | |
| | | | |
| | | | |
| | | | |
| | | | |

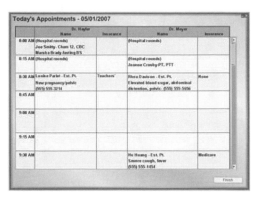

• Now click again on any patient in the patient list. Then on the office map, click on **Reception**. At the Reception desk, click on **Today's Appointments** to view the day's schedule. Look for each patient's name and note next to his or her name on the table in question 1 whether that patient is a new patient (NP) or an established patient (Est. Pt.) (*Note:* You will return to fill in the remaining columns of the table later in this exercise.)

*Click on Today's Appointments.*

2. With the schedule of Today's Appointments still open, make a list below of the patients Dr. Hayler is to see in the morning. Place these patients in the correct order for their appointments and note whether the medical record can be pulled from the files of established patients or whether a new record should be prepared.

3. What medical records will need to be pulled from the files for Dr. Meyer's morning patients? Will any of these patients need to have a new record prepared? List these patients and their record needs below (in the order of their appointment times).

• Click **Finish** to close the appointment book and return to the Reception desk.
• Click the exit arrow in right lower corner of screen.

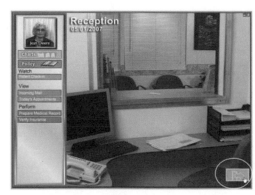

*Click the exit arrow.*

• From the Summary Menu, click on **Return to Map**; then click **Yes** to return to the office map and select another patient.

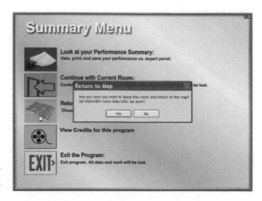

*Click on Return to Map. When prompted, click Yes.*

• Beginning with the first patient on the left in the patient list, open each patient's chart, click on the **Patient Medical Information** tab, and select **Progress Notes**. Based on what you find, record the patients' first and last dates of service in columns 2 and 4 in the table in question 1. (*Note:* New patients will not have any forms in their chart. Use today's virtual date—5-1-07—as their first date of service; there will be no "last date of service" for new patients.)

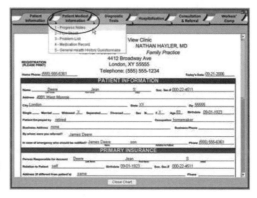

*Click on Progress Notes and find the first and last dates of service.*

• When you have recorded the date(s) for the first patient, click **Close Chart**; then click the exit arrow.
• From the Summary Menu, click on **Return to Map**.
• Select your next patient, open the chart, and record the date(s) in the table.
• Continue these steps for each patient until you have completed the table in question 1.

4. Using the table in question 1 as a reference, list the patients' names in alphabetic order in the left column below. In the right column indicate whether the medical records for each patient will be available in the file cabinet of established patients or whether the record will have to be organized and placed in the correct position as a new medical record

| Alphabetic List of Patients | New or Established Record? |
| --- | --- |
| | |

5. As you pull the medical records for established patients, you will need to change the year on the medical records for these patients (unless the patient has already been seen in the current year). List the established patients below and indicate what year will need to be relabeled on their medical record (if this applies).

| Name of Established Patient | Year That Will Need to Be Relabeled |
| --- | --- |
| | |

6. At the end of the morning, the medical records need to be filed correctly to prevent loss and to ensure proper time management. Below, list in alphabetic order the names of patients who had morning appointments today and whose records will need to be refiled.

7. Which of the following would not be used to help prevent misfiling of medical records?
   a. Colored letter tabs for use with names
   b. Colored tabs for the last year seen in office
   c. Outguides
   d. Alphabet tabs in the filing system

8. The two filing systems most often used in a medical office are _____ and

   _____ filing.

# 9

# Insurance Forms and Verification

---

**Reading Assignment:** Chapter 17—Basics of Diagnostic Coding
Chapter 18—Basics of Procedural Coding
Chapter 19—The Health Insurance Claim Form
Chapter 20—Third Party Reimbursement

**Patients:** Shaunti Begay, Louise Parlet, John R. Simmons, Janet Jones

## Objectives:

- Apply managed care policies and procedures to office billing and coding.
- Use third party guidelines for preparing insurance claims and collecting co-payments.
- Perform procedural coding.
- Perform diagnostic coding.
- Prepare a clean insurance claim form.

## Overview:

In this lesson you will perform the necessary steps for preparing a clean claim for insurance purposes and collecting co-payments that are due to the practice. Completing these steps requires the correct use of managed care policies and procedures and the proper application of the office Policy Manual. A clean claim includes the appropriate diagnostic and procedural codes, as well as the proper completion of the insurance claim form.

### Exercise 1

  **CD-ROM Activity—Verifying Insurance for a New Patient**

30 minutes

- Sign in to Mountain View Clinic.
- From the patient list, select **Shaunti Begay**.

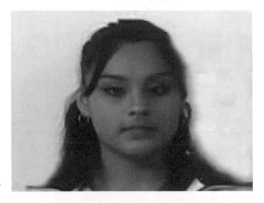

*Shaunti Begay*

- On the office map, highlight and click on **Reception**.

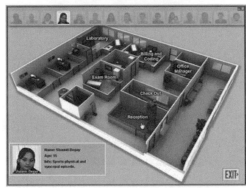

*Click on Reception.*

- At the Reception desk, click on **Policy** to open the office Policy Manual.

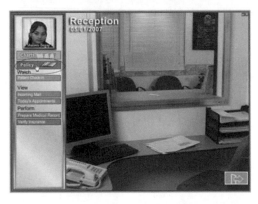

*Click on Policy.*

- Type "17" in the search bar and click the magnifying glass once. This will take you to page 17 of the Policy Manual. Scroll up to adjust the page and read the policies that apply when patients have insurance coverage that is not accepted by the medical practice.

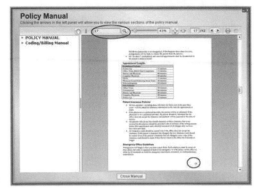

*Search for page 17.*

1. According to the Policy Manual, what information should be obtained from the patient when the appointment is made?

2. Why is it important for the medical assistant to verify *at the time the appointment is made* whether the office is a preferred provider with the patient's insurance?

→ • Scroll up to page 14 of the Policy Manual and read the section on Telephone Policies.

3. What does the Policy Manual state about collecting payments, co-pays, and percentages of charges for patient visits?

→ • Click **Close Manual** to return to the Reception desk.
   • Click on **Patient Check-In** to view the video of Shaunti's arrival at the clinic.

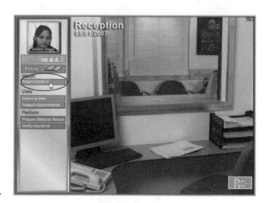

*Click on Patient Check-In.*

• At the end of the video, click **Close** to return to the Reception desk.

→ • At the Reception desk, click on **Verify Insurance** to obtain the required information for Shaunti's visit.

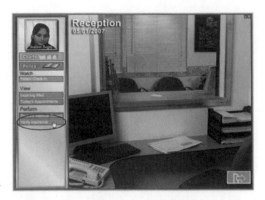

*Click on Verify Insurance.*

• Select the appropriate question to ask Shaunti regarding her insurance; then review the Insurance Cards on the next screen.

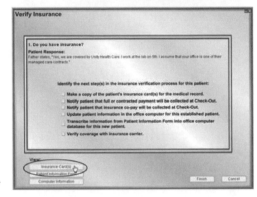

*Review the Insurance Cards.*

• Click **Finish** to return to the Reception desk.
• Click again on **Policy** to reopen the Policy Manual.
• From the menu on the left side of the screen, click on the arrow next to **Coding/Billing Manual** to view the additional headings for that section of the Policy Manual.
• Click the arrow next to **Financial Policy** and select **Accepted Insurance Carriers** from the list.

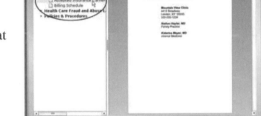

*Click Accepted Insurance Carriers.*

• Click **Close Manual** to return to the Reception desk.

4. Was Kristin correct in stating that Mountain View Clinic was not a participating provider for Shaunti's insurance plan?

5. What did Shaunti's mother say about the information she gave the receptionist regarding their insurance coverage when she made the appointment?

6. What steps should the medical assistant have taken to avoid the confusion that occurred when Shaunti checked in?

 • Click the exit arrow to leave the Reception desk.
• From the Summary Menu, select **Return to Map**.

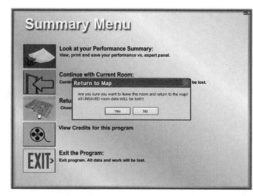

*Click Return to Map.*

### Exercise 2

 ### CD-ROM Activity—Obtaining a Referral for an Established Patient

 30 minutes

• Select **Louise Parlet** from the patient list. (*Note:* If you have exited the program, sign in again to Mountain View Clinic and select Louise Parlet from the patient list.)

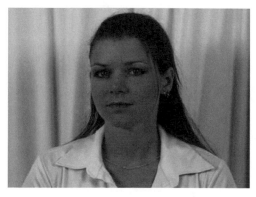

*Louise Parlet*

➤ • On the office map, highlight and click on **Check Out**.

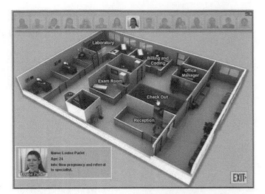

*Click on Check Out.*

• At the desk, click on **Patient Check-Out** to view the video.

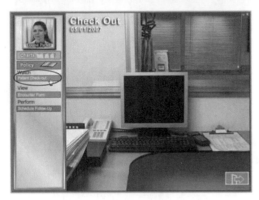

*Click on Patient Check-Out.*

• At the end of the video, click **Close** to return to the desk.

1. Why is it important that the medical assistant assist Ms. Parlet in obtaining approval from her insurance company for the referral to Dr. Lockett?

2. After receiving the precertification verification number, how should the medical assistant handle the verification number?

- Next, click on **Charts** to open Ms. Parlet's medical record.
- Under the **Patient Medical Information** tab, select **3-Progress Notes** and read Dr. Hayler's notes regarding the examination.

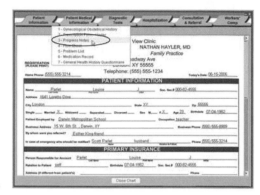

*Click on 3-Progress Notes.*

3. What instructions does Dr. Hayler give about the results of the lab work? How do these instructions affect the insurance coverage?

- Click **Close Chart** to return to the Check Out desk.
- Click the exit arrow; from the Summary Menu, select **Return to Map**.

### Exercise 3

 **CD-ROM Activity—Coding an Office Visit of a New Adult Patient**

 30 minutes

- Select **John R. Simmons** from the patient list. (*Note:* If you have exited the program, sign in again to Mountain View Clinic and select John R. Simmons from the patient list.)

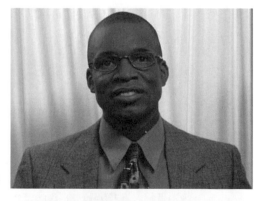

*John R. Simmons*

- On the office map, highlight and click on **Billing and Coding**.

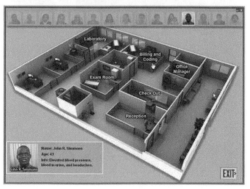

*Click on Billing and Coding.*

• At the Billing and Coding desk, click on **Encounter Form** to view the diagnostic and procedural information for Dr. Simmons' visit.

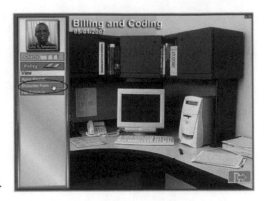

*Click on Encounter Form.*

1. In the ICD-9 section of the Encounter Form, which diagnoses are checked off for Dr. Simmons' visit?

2. Which of these diagnoses should receive an ICD-9 code? If there are any diagnoses that should not be coded, explain why not.

3. When should the home-obtained hemoccult testing be billed and coded? Explain your answer.

 • Click **Finish** to close the Encounter Form and return to the Billing and Coding desk.
   • Click on **Charts** to open Dr. Simmons' medical record and select **5-Insurance Cards** from under the **Patient Information** tab.

4. Using the information on the insurance cards found in the medical record, what is the co-pay on the patient's insurance? What is the payment rate on the secondary insurance?

5. What is meant by PCP?

6. What is meant by POS?

- Click **Close Chart** to return to the Billing and Coding desk.
- Click the exit arrow; from the Summary Menu, select **Return to Map**.

### Exercise 4

### CD-ROM Activity—Insurance Versus Workers' Compensation Claims

15 minutes

- From the patient list, select **Janet Jones**. (*Note:* If you have exited the program, sign in again to Mountain View Clinic and select Janet Jones from the patient list.)

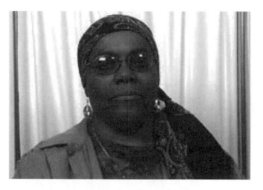

*Janet Jones*

- On the office map, highlight and click on **Billing and Coding**.

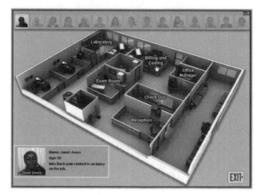

*Click on Billing and Coding.*

- Click on **Charts** to open Janet Jones' medical record.
- Next, click on the **Patient Information** tab.

1.  You will notice that in Ms. Jones' medical record, there is no information about private insurance coverage. Why is this important for this case?

2.  What information is needed for a Workers' Compensation claim that is not needed for a private insurance claim?

➡ •   Now click on the tab labeled **Workers' Comp**.

3.  What information do you find under this tab in Ms. Jones' medical record?

4.  If the Workers' Compensation carrier declares Ms. Jones' claim to be nonindustrial and refuses to pay it, is Mountain View Clinic required to write off the balance?

# LESSON 10 ——————————

# Bookkeeping

———————————————————

**Patients:** All

**Objectives:**

- Post daily entries on the day sheet and prepare bank deposits at the end of the day.
- Process credit balances, NSF checks, and checks from collection agencies.
- Perform billing and collections procedures.
- Process credit balances and complete necessary steps to process a refund, including preparation of a check.
- Reconcile a bank statement.
- Maintain a petty cash fund.
- Discuss the maintenance of records for accounting and banking purposes.
- Discuss the importance of managing accounts payable promptly.

**Overview:**

In this lesson the basic bookkeeping procedures will be accomplished. All patients will be added to the day sheet, along with the payments and the NSF check received in today's mail. A deposit record will be prepared. The steps for reconciliation of the bank statement and maintenance of records for accounting purposes will also be covered.

### Exercise 1

  **CD-ROM Activity—Posting Charges to Ledger Cards**

30 minutes

- Sign in to Mountain View Clinic.
- Select **Jade Wong** from the patient list.

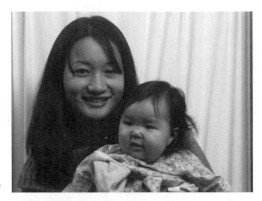

*Jade Wong*

- On the office map, highlight and click on **Billing and Coding**.

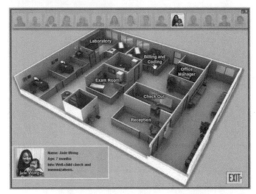

*Click on Billing and Coding.*

- In the Billing and Coding office, select **Encounter Form** to review the services that will be billed for Jade's visit.

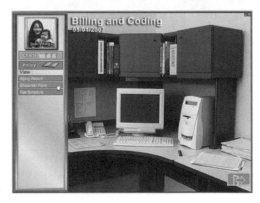

*Select Encounter Form.*

1. a. Using the Encounter Form for Jade Wong, begin completing the blank ledger card below.
   b. In the column marked Professional Service, list each individual service provided, but do not enter any fee or balance information.
   c. After the last service has been entered, be sure to record that the co-pay was collected and enter the amount in the Payment column.

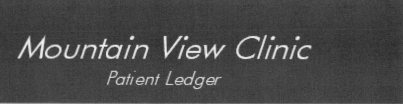

Patient Name:
Insurance Type:

| Date | Professional Service | Fee ($) | Payment ($) | Adj. ($) | Prev. Bal. ($) | New Balance ($) |
|------|----------------------|---------|-------------|----------|----------------|-----------------|
|  |  |  |  |  |  |  |
|  |  |  |  |  |  |  |
|  |  |  |  |  |  |  |
|  |  |  |  |  |  |  |
|  |  |  |  |  |  |  |
|  |  |  |  |  |  |  |
|  |  |  |  |  |  |  |
|  |  |  |  |  |  |  |
|  |  |  |  |  |  |  |
|  |  |  |  |  |  |  |
|  |  |  |  |  |  |  |
|  |  |  |  |  |  |  |
|  |  |  |  |  |  |  |
|  |  |  |  |  |  |  |
|  |  |  |  |  |  |  |
|  |  |  |  |  |  |  |
| Totals |  |  |  |  |  |  |

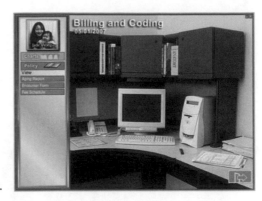

- Click **Finish** to return to Billing and Coding.
- Now click on **Fee Schedule** to review the amount Mountain View Clinic charges for various services and procedures.

*Click on Fee Schedule.*

- Again using the ledger card on the previous page, fill in the fees charged for the listed services and calculate the balances. (*Note:* The balance should be adjusted line by line as each service or payment is added or subtracted.)

2. After filling in the services, charges, and payments for Jade's current visit, should the ledger card be totaled as indicated at the bottom of the card? Explain your answer.

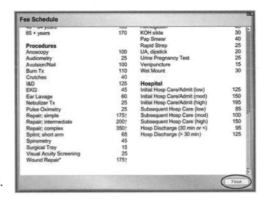

- Click **Finish** to close the Fee Schedule; then click the exit arrow to leave Billing and Coding.

*Click Finish.*

- On the Summary Menu, click on **Return to Map** and continue to the next exercise.

**Exercise 2**

 **CD-ROM Activity—Posting Entries to a Day Sheet**

 60 minutes

1. In this activity you will post charges and payments for the patients who were seen in the office today.
   a. In the Patient Name column on the blank day sheet on the next page, list the patients in the following order: Jade Wong, Louise Parlet, Hu Huang, Rhea Davison, Jesus Santo, Jean Deere, Tristan Tsosie, Wilson Metcalf, Renee Anderson, Jose Imero, Shaunti Begay, Janet Jones, Kevin McKinzie, John R. Simmons, and Teresa Hernandez.
   b. Select Jade Wong from the patient list. Then click on **Check Out** on the office map. Once in the Check Out area, open the **Encounter Form**.
   c. Using one line per patient, complete each column on the day sheet using the Total Charges, Previous Balance, and Amount Received information listed on the Encounter Form. Refer back to the ledger card in Exercise 1 to confirm your totals. (*Note:* Unlike the ledger card, the Professional Service column on the day sheet is a summary description of the visit.)
   d. For the purposes of this exercise, also make a note next to each patient's name to indicate whether the patient paid by cash, check, or credit card. If payment was made by check, include the check number.
   e. Repeat the above steps by selecting each patient and opening his or her Encounter Form at Check Out. As you finish each patient's portion of the day sheet, click **Finish** to close the Encounter Form. Click the exit arrow to leave Check Out and **Return to Map** to select the next patient.
   f. When you finish recording the information for the last patient on the list, remain at the office map to continue with the next question.

# Mountain View Clinic
## Daysheet

| Date | Professional Service | Fee | Payment | Adjustment | New Balance | Old Balance | Patient's Name | Distribution Dr. Hayler | Distribution Dr. Meyer |
|------|---------------------|-----|---------|------------|-------------|-------------|----------------|------------------------|------------------------|
|      |                     |     |         |            |             |             |                |                        |                        |
|      |                     |     |         |            |             |             |                |                        |                        |
|      |                     |     |         |            |             |             |                |                        |                        |
|      |                     |     |         |            |             |             |                |                        |                        |
|      |                     |     |         |            |             |             |                |                        |                        |
|      |                     |     |         |            |             |             |                |                        |                        |
|      |                     |     |         |            |             |             |                |                        |                        |
|      |                     |     |         |            |             |             |                |                        |                        |
|      |                     |     |         |            |             |             |                |                        |                        |
|      |                     |     |         |            |             |             |                |                        |                        |
| TOTALS |                   |     |         |            |             |             |                |                        |                        |

• From the office map, click on **Reception**. (The selected patient should be Teresa Hernandez, the last patient on the list in question 1.)
• At the Reception desk, click on **Incoming Mail** to view the day's correspondence.

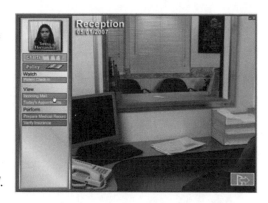

*Click Incoming Mail.*

2. a. View each piece of incoming mail; then on the blank day sheet on the next page, record any payments *received* by the clinic and any charges *paid* by the clinic in the appropriate columns.
   b. Be sure to include a description of the payment/charge and the patient's name.
   c. For the purposes of this exercise, make a note of the bank and check number next to the name of any patient who paid by check.
   d. To complete the remaining columns, first click **Finish** to close the mail.
   e. Next, click the exit arrow and **Return to Map**.
   f. Click on **Office Manager** and then on **Day Sheet** (under View) to find any previous balance information. Then recalculate the balance and record in the New Balance column.

# Mountain View Clinic
## Daysheet

| Distribution | | Patient's Name | Old Balance | New Balance | Adjustment | Payment | Fee | Professional Service | Date |
|---|---|---|---|---|---|---|---|---|---|
| Dr. Meyer | Dr. Hayler | | | | | | | | |
| | | | | | | | | | |
| | | | | | | | | | |
| | | | | | | | | | |
| | | | | | | | | | |
| | | | | | | | | | |
| TOTALS | | | | | | | TOTALS | | |

• Click **Finish** and continue to the next exercise.

### Exercise 3

 **Writing Activity—Preparing a Bank Deposit**

 15 minutes

1. Using the information recorded in completed day sheets in Exercise 2, you will now prepare a bank deposit (both front and back) for the accounts receivable for the day. Be sure the total on the deposit slip balances with the total of receivables on the day sheet.

    Below, complete the front side of the deposit slip.

**DEPOSIT SLIP**

Clarion National Bank
90 Grape Vine Road
London, XY  55555-0001

*Mountain View Clinic*
*4412 Broadway*
*London, XY 55555*

Date: _____

_____
SIGN HERE IN TELLER'S PRESENCE FOR CASH RECEIVED

| CASH | | | TOTAL |
|---|---|---|---|
| | Currency | $ | |
| | Coin | $ | |
| | Total Cash | | $ |
| CHECKS | See other side for detail | | $ |
| - CASH REC'D | | | $ |
| NET DEPOSIT | | | $ |

2. Below, complete the back portion of the bank deposit slip. (*Note:* The bank number cannot be obtained from the day sheet. For the purposes of this exercise, use the check number as a substitute.)

## BANK DEPOSIT DETAIL

PAYMENTS

| BANK NUMBER | BY CHECK OR PMO | BY COIN OR CURRENCY | CREDIT CARD | |
|---|---|---|---|---|
| | | | | |
| | | | | |
| | | | | |
| | | | | |
| | | | | |
| | | | | |
| | | | | |
| | | | | |
| | | | | |
| | | | | |
| | | | | |
| | | | | |
| | | | | |
| | | | | |
| | | | | |
| | | | | |
| | | | | |
| | | | | |
| | | | | |
| **TOTALS** | | | | |
| CURRENCY | | | | |
| COIN | | | | |
| CHECKS | | | | |
| CREDIT CARDS | | | | |
| TOTAL RECEIPTS | | | | |
| LESS CREDIT CARD $ | | | | |
| **TOTAL DEPOSIT** | | | | |
| DEPOSIT DATE _____ | | | | |

**Exercise 4**

 **CD-ROM Activity—Processing Credit Balances**

 20 minutes

- Remain in the manager's office and click on **Day Sheet**. (*Note:* If you have exited the manager's office and are at the office map, click on **Office Manager** and then click on **Day Sheet**.)

  1. Two patients listed on the day sheet have overpaid, resulting in a credit balance. What are the names of these two patients, and how much money should be refunded to each of them?

  2. The day sheet indicates that _____ has already been sent a refund, but the refund for _____ still needs to be processed.

  3. Using the blank check below, process the outstanding refund for payment.

| 173975 | | |
|---|---|---|
| DATE:_____ | | |
| TO: _____ | | |
| FOR: _____ | | |
| BALANCE BROUGHT FORWARD | | |
| DEPOSITS | | |
| BALANCE | | |
| AMT THIS CHECK | | |
| BALANCE CARRIED FORWARD | | |

MOUNTAIN VIEW CLINIC                173975
4412 Broadway
London, XY 55555                    94-72/1224

                        Date: _____

Pay to the order of: _____

_____ Dollars

Clarion National Bank
        Member FDIC
90 Grape Vine Road                  _____
London, XY 55555-0001                   Authorized Signature

  ||⑈ 005509 ||⑈  446782011 ||⑈  678800470

 - Click **Finish** to return to the manager's office.

### Exercise 5

 **CD-ROM Activity—Maintaining Petty Cash Fund**

 30 minutes

- In the office manager's office, click on **Petty Cash**. (*Note:* If you have exited the manager's office and are at the office map, click on **Office Manager** and select **Petty Cash**.)

1. Petty cash was used to pay for the mailing of a certified letter. What is the receipt number and date from this transaction?

2. On 5-1-07, the administrative medical assistant was asked to obtain soft drinks for an office celebration to be held that afternoon. These were bought at Sav-A-Grocery for the amount of $24.56. She also mailed a large package at the post office. The cost for mailing the package was $15.08. Using the form below, fill out the first petty cash voucher.

Date: _____     No.: ___109___

Amount: [        ]

### PETTY CASH VOUCHER

For: _____

Charge to: _____

_____

Approved by:                          Received by:

_____          _____

*Authorized Signature*

3. Now fill out the second petty cash voucher.

Date: _____            No.: _110_

Amount: [        ]

PETTY CASH VOUCHER

For: _____

Charge to: _____
_____

Approved by:                    Received by:

_____          _____
*Authorized Signature*

4. Using the completed petty cash vouchers from questions 2 and 3, update the petty cash log below accordingly. Be sure to distribute the expenses to the proper expense column.

| NO. | DATE | DESCRIPTION | AMOUNT | OFFICE EXP. | AUTO. | MISC. | BALANCE |
|---|---|---|---|---|---|---|---|
|  | 2/16/2007 | Fund Established (check #217) |  |  |  |  | 200.00 |
| 101 | 2/24/2007 | Certified Letter | 3.74 | 3.74 |  |  | 196.26 |
| 102 | 3/1/2007 | Staff Meeting/Lunch | 24.60 |  |  | 24.60 | 171.66 |
| 103 | 3/6/2007 | Coffee | 4.32 |  |  | 4.32 | 167.34 |
| 104 | 3/8/2007 | Tympanic Thermometer | 38.00 | 38.00 |  |  | 129.34 |
| 105 | 3/8/2007 | Parking Fee | 6.00 |  | 6.00 |  | 123.34 |
| 106 | 4/1/2007 | Staff Meeting/Lunch | 27.43 |  |  | 27.43 | 95.91 |
| 107 | 4/13/2007 | Miscellaneous Supplies | 9.01 | 9.01 |  |  | 86.90 |
| 108 | 4/21/2007 | Patient Birthday Cards | 12.17 | 12.17 |  |  | 74.73 |

5. Office policy states that petty cash should be replenished when the amount falls below $50. Use the blank check below to replenish the petty cash fund to the full $200 balance as required by the office policy. Then, using the updated petty cash log in question 4, verify the petty cash fund balances by totaling all the columns, and add this transaction to the log.

| 173976 | MOUNTAIN VIEW CLINIC<br>4412 Broadway<br>London, XY 55555 | 173976 |
|---|---|---|
| DATE:_____ | | 94-721/224 |
| TO: _____ | | Date: _____ |
| FOR: _____ | Pay to the order of: _____ | |
| ACCOUNT NO. _____ | _____ Dollars | |
| AMOUNT PAID    $ | Clarion National Bank<br>Member FDIC<br>90 Grape Vine Road<br>London, XY 55555-0001 | _____<br>Authorized Signature |

||∎ 005503 ||∎ 446782011 ||∎ 678800470

 • Click **Finish** to return to the manager's office.
  • Click the exit arrow; from the Summary Menu, select **Return to Map**.
  • On the office map, select **Jose Imero** from the patient list and click on **Check Out**.
  • At the Check Out desk, select **Patient Check Out** (under Watch) to view the video.

6. What are the ethical implications of Kristin asking another medical assistant for money from petty cash?

  • Click **Close** to return to the Check Out desk.
  • Click the exit arrow; from the Summary Menu, select **Return to Map**.

### Exercise 6

  **CD-ROM Activity—Managing Accounts Payable**

30 minutes

- Using any patient from the patient list, click on **Reception** on the office map. (*Note:* You may continue with Jose Imero from the previous exercise.)
- Select **Incoming Mail** (under View) and review pieces 8 and 9.

1. Indicate whether each of the following statements is true or false.

   a. _____ When accounts payable arrive, the date for payment with discounts should be noted.

   b. _____ It really does not matter what day of the month an accounts payable payment is made, as long as it is paid before the next billing cycle.

   c. _____ Invoices should be marked with the date and check number, as well as the initials of the person preparing the check.

   d. _____ All accounts payables should be checked against invoices and packing slips before payment is made.

   e. _____ All vendors will present invoices before payment is due.

2. Which of the following information does the accounts payable person need to correctly process and post the payment of the invoices (pieces 8 and 9 of the incoming mail)? Select all that apply.

   _____ Invoice number

   _____ Company name

   _____ Name of customer service representative

   _____ Date of check

   _____ Account number

   _____ Company address

   _____ Company phone number

   _____ Name of the company's bank

   _____ Company's bank account number

   _____ Type of expense

   _____ Amount of the check

   _____ Invoice date

   _____ Check number

• Click **Finish** to close the mail and return to the Reception desk.
• Click the exit arrow; from the Summary Menu, select **Return to Map**.

### Exercise 7

 CD-ROM Activity—Reconciling a Bank Statement

 30 minutes

In today's mail, the clinic's bank statement arrives. This is found in the manager's office. She is extremely busy and asks that you take the time to reconcile the statement for her.

• On the office map, click on **Office Manager** to enter the manager's office. (*Note:* For this task, it does not matter which patient is selected. You may continue with Jose Imero from the previous exercise.)
• From the menu on the left, select **Bank Statement**.

1. a. Using the check ledger below, review the bank statement and check off each deposit, check, withdrawal, ATM transaction, or credit listed on the statement.
   b. If the statement shows any interest paid to the account, any service charges, bank fees, automatic payments, or ATM transactions withdrawn from the account that are not listed on the check ledger, make an entry for those items now and recalculate the account balance in the ledger.

| No. | Date | Description | Payment/ Debit | Ref | Deposit/ Credit | Balance |
|---|---|---|---|---|---|---|
| 1216 | 3/5/2007 | Rocke Medical | $625.00 | | | $9,264.35 |
| 1217 | 3/5/2007 | Wal Store | $38.46 | | | $9,225.89 |
| 1218 | 3/6/2007 | Lorenz Equipment | $1,006.00 | | | $8,219.89 |
| 1219 | 3/8/2007 | Office Station | $199.43 | | | $8,020.46 |
| | 3/10/2007 | Dep. Daily Trans | | | $1,050.00 | $10,833.46 |
| 1220 | 3/10/2007 | West Electric | $93.99 | | | $7,926.47 |
| | 3/12/2007 | Dep. Daily Trans | | | $2,008.00 | $9,934.47 |
| 1221 | 3/12/2007 | Office Depot | $102.01 | | | $9,832.46 |
| 1222 | 3/12/2007 | Video Inc. | $49.00 | | | $9,783.46 |
| | 3/15/2007 | Dep. Daily Trans | | | $1,002.00 | $11,835.46 |
| 1223 | 3/17/2007 | Bonus | $200.00 | | | $12,560.46 |
| 1224 | 3/17/2007 | Bonus | $200.00 | | | $12,360.46 |
| 1225 | 3/17/2007 | Bonus | $200.00 | | | $12,160.46 |
| | 3/20/2007 | Dep. Daily Trans | | | $925.00 | $12,760.46 |
| 1226 | 3/21/2007 | Jamison Medical | $2,024.20 | | | $10,136.26 |
| 1227 | 3/22/2007 | Healthy Living Magazine | $32.95 | | | $10,103.31 |
| 1228 | 3/22/2007 | Greater London Electric | $422.00 | | | $9,681.31 |
| 1229 | 3/24/2007 | Office Station | $344.70 | | | $9,336.61 |
| 1230 | 3/25/2007 | Summer Oxygen | $230.99 | | | $9,105.62 |
| | 3/27/2007 | Dep. Daily Trans | | | $1,550.00 | $10,655.62 |
| | | | | | | |
| | | | | | | |
| | | | | | | |
| | | | | | | |
| | | | | | | |
| | | | | | | |

2. Now complete the bank reconciliation worksheet below.

**THIS WORKSHEET IS PROVIDED TO HELP YOU BALANCE YOUR ACCOUNT**

1. Go through your register and mark each check, withdrawal, Express ATM transaction, payment, deposit or other credit listed on your statement. Be sure that your register shows any interest paid into your account, and any service charges, bank fees, automatic payments, or Express Transfers withdrawn from your account during this statement period.

2. Using the chart below, list any outstanding checks, Express ATM withdrawals, payments or any other withdrawals (including any from previous months) that are listed in your register but are not shown on this statement.

3. Balance your account by filling in the spaces below.

| ITEMS OUTSTANDING | | |
|---|---|---|
| NUMBER | AMOUNT | |
| | | |
| | | |
| | | |
| | | |
| | | |
| | | |
| | | |
| | | |
| | | |
| | | |
| | | |
| | | |
| | | |
| | | |
| | | |
| | | |
| | | |
| | | |
| | | |
| | | |
| | | |
| | | |
| | | |
| **TOTAL** | | |

**ENTER**

The NEW BALANCE shown on this statement ------------------------------- $ _____ __

**ADD**

Any deposits listed in your register or      $ _____ __
transfers into your account which are        $ _____ __
not shown on this statement                  $ _____ __
                                            +$ _____ __

TOTAL------------------------------------+ $ _____ __

**CALCULATE THE SUBTOTAL** ------------------------------------- $ _____ __

**SUBTRACT**

The total outstanding checks and
Withdrawals from the chart at the left -------------------------------------------- $ _____ __

**CALCULATE THE ENDING BALANCE**

This amount should be the same as
The current balance shown in your
Check register -------------------------------------------------------------- $ _____ __

**Exercise 8**

 **Writing Activity—Maintaining Financial Records**

15 minutes

1. Indicate whether each of the following statements is true or false.

    a. _____ All financial records may be discarded after 7 years.

    b. _____ If financial records are discarded early, legal implications are possible.

    c. _____ All financial records should be kept in an active file for 7 years.

    d. _____ The office Policy Manual should provide the guidelines for record retention.

    e. _____ When financial records are stored, the storage boxes should be labeled and stored in logical order.

    f. _____ The medical assistant should obtain the physician's permission before destroying any records.

    g. _____ All financial records must be maintained for the same time limit.

# Payroll Proecedures

/⦾⦾ **Reading Assignment:**  Chapter 23—Management of Practice Finances
  • Payroll Records

**Patients:**  None

**Objectives:**

• Describe steps necessary in preparing payroll.
• Process employee payroll.

**Overview:**

For administrative medical assistants, the task of preparing an employee payroll may be a routine function. This lesson will give you practice in preparing payroll for employees.

### Exercise 1

  **CD-ROM Activity—Processing Payroll**

15 minutes

- Sign in to Mountain View Clinic.
- On the office map, highlight and click on **Office Manager** to enter the manager's office. (*Note:* You do not need to select a patient for this exercise.)

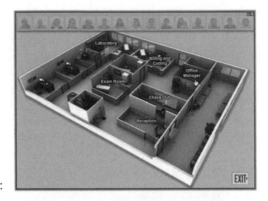

*Click on Office Manager.*

- Click on **Payroll Forms** to view the office payroll records.

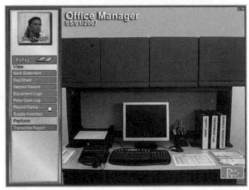

*Click on Payroll Forms.*

- The time sheet for employee Cathy Wright will appear first. Review and confirm that the number of hours have been calculated correctly.
- Next, click on the down arrow next to Person and select **Susan Bronski**.

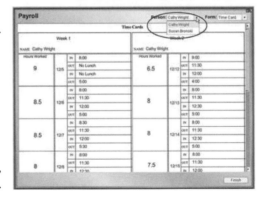

*To change employees, click on the down arrow next to the name.*

- Review Susan Bronski's time sheet and confirm the calculations for the number of hours she worked.

  1. Cathy Wright's total number of hours worked: _____

     Susan Bronski's total number of hours worked: _____

2. Cathy Wright has been employed by the clinic for 10 years. Her salary is $18.00 per hour for the first 80 hours and $27.00 per hour for any hours over 80 during the 2-week pay period. Compute the gross pay for Cathy for the 2-week period.

3. Susan Bronski is a relatively new employee who is making $15.00 per hour for the first 80 hours and $20 per hour for hours over 80. Complete the gross pay for Susan for the 2-week period.

 • Now review the W-4 form filled out by each employee.

• To view Cathy Wright's W-4 form, first make sure her name is selected from the drop-down menu next to Person. Next, click on the down arrow next to Form and select **W-4**. Review her form.

• To view Susan Bronski's W-4 form, select her name from the drop-down menu next to Person.

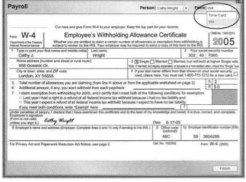

*Click the arrow next to Form and select W-4.*

4. Cathy Wright elected to have her federal taxes withheld under which designation?

_____   Single

_____   Married

_____   Married, but withhold at the higher single rate

5. The number of allowances claimed by Cathy Wright is _____.

6. Did Cathy Wright elect to have any additional money withheld from her paycheck for federal taxes? If yes, how much?

7. Susan Bronski will have her federal taxes withheld under which designation?

_____ Single

_____ Married

_____ Married, but withhold at the higher single rate

8. The number of allowances claimed by Susan Bronski is _____.

9. Did Susan Bronski elect to have any additional money withheld from her paycheck for federal taxes? If yes, how much?

**Exercise 2**

**Writing Activity—Calculating Net Pay**

15 minutes

1.

## Table 5. Percentage Method—2007 Amount for One Withholding Allowance

| Payroll Period | One Withholding Allowance |
|---|---|
| Weekly | $    65.38 |
| Biweekly | 130.77 |
| Semimonthly | 141.67 |
| Monthly | 283.33 |
| Quarterly | 850.00 |
| Semiannually | 1,700.00 |
| Annually | 3,400.00 |
| Daily or miscellaneous (each day of the payroll period) | 13.08 |

Using the above table and the number of allowances each employee designated on her W-4, calculate the total withholding allowance for Cathy Wright and Susan Bronski.

Total withholding allowance for Cathy Wright: _____

Total withholding allowance for Susan Bronski: _____

2. Now subtract the total withholding allowance from each employee's gross pay to calculate the adjusted gross pay.

Cathy Wright's adjusted gross pay: _____

Susan Bronski's adjusted gross pay: _____

3. Below is the table for calculating the appropriate federal income tax withholding for Cathy Wright and Susan Bronski, using the percentage method.

## TABLE 2—BIWEEKLY Payroll Period

| (a) SINGLE person (including head of household)— | | | (b) MARRIED person— | | |
|---|---|---|---|---|---|
| If the amount of wages (after subtracting withholding allowances) is: | The amount of income tax to withhold is: | | If the amount of wages (after subtracting withholding allowances) is: | The amount of income tax to withhold is: | |
| Not over $102 . . . . | $0 | | Not over $308 . . . . | $0 | |
| Over—  But not over— | | of excess over— | Over—  But not over— | | of excess over— |
| $102    —$389 . . | 10% | —$102 | $308    —$898 . . | 10% | —$308 |
| $389    —$1,289 . . | $28.70 plus 15% | —$389 | $898    —$2,719 . . | $59.00 plus 15% | —$898 |
| $1,289  —$2,964 . . | $163.70 plus 25% | —$1,289 | $2,719  —$5,146 . . | $332.15 plus 25% | —$2,719 |
| $2,964  —$6,262 . . | $582.45 plus 28% | —$2,964 | $5,146  —$7,813 . . | $938.90 plus 28% | —$5,146 |
| $6,262  —$13,525 . . | $1,505.89 plus 33% | —$6,262 | $7,813  —$13,731 . . | $1,685.66 plus 33% | —$7,813 |
| $13,525 . . . . . . | $3,902.68 plus 35% | —$13,525 | $13,731 . . . . . . | $3,638.60 plus 35% | —$13,731 |

a. Using the information in the table above, calculate the amount of federal income tax that will be withheld for Cathy Wright.

b. Account for the following additional deductions:
Medicare = 1.45%
Social Security = 6.2%
Health Insurance = $125 per pay
State Income Tax = 1%
Retirement Plan = $150 per pay

| | |
|---|---|
| **Federal Income Tax** | |
| **Medicare** | |
| **Social Security** | |
| **Health Insurance** | |
| **State Income Tax** | |
| **Retirement Plan** | |

4. What is the net pay for Cathy Wright?

5.

## TABLE 2—BIWEEKLY Payroll Period

| (a) SINGLE person (including head of household)— | | | | (b) MARRIED person— | | | |
|---|---|---|---|---|---|---|---|
| If the amount of wages (after subtracting withholding allowances) is: | | The amount of income tax to withhold is: | | If the amount of wages (after subtracting withholding allowances) is: | | The amount of income tax to withhold is: | |
| Not over $102 . . . . . | | $0 | | Not over $308 . . . . . | | $0 | |
| Over— | But not over— | | of excess over— | Over— | But not over— | | of excess over— |
| $102 | —$389 . . | 10% | —$102 | $308 | —$898 . . | 10% | —$308 |
| $389 | —$1,289 . . | $28.70 plus 15% | —$389 | $898 | —$2,719 . . | $59.00 plus 15% | —$898 |
| $1,289 | —$2,964 . . | $163.70 plus 25% | —$1,289 | $2,719 | —$5,146 . . | $332.15 plus 25% | —$2,719 |
| $2,964 | —$6,262 . . | $582.45 plus 28% | —$2,964 | $5,146 | —$7,813 . . | $938.90 plus 28% | —$5,146 |
| $6,262 | —$13,525 . . | $1,505.89 plus 33% | —$6,262 | $7,813 | —$13,731 . . | $1,685.66 plus 33% | —$7,813 |
| $13,525 | . . . . . . | $3,902.68 plus 35% | —$13,525 | $13,731 | . . . . . . | $3,638.60 plus 35% | —$13,731 |

a. Using the information in the table above, calculate the amount of federal income tax that will be withheld for Susan Bronski, who will filed as head of household.

b. Account for the following additional deductions:
Medicare = 1.45%
Social Security = 6.2%
Health Insurance = $175 per pay
State Income Tax = 1%
Savings Plan = $50 per pay
Additional Tax Withholding from W-4 = $190.00

| Federal Income Tax | |
|---|---|
| Medicare | |
| Social Security | |
| Health Insurance | |
| State Income Tax | |
| Retirement Plan | |

6. What is the net pay for Susan Bronski?

**Exercise 3**

## CD-ROM Activity—Writing the Check for Payroll

15 minutes

1. You are now ready to prepare and issue the payroll checks for Cathy Wright and Susan Bronski. To obtain the correct ending date for the pay period, return to the employees' time sheets by clicking on **Payroll Forms** in the manager's office. Date the checks for the Monday following the end of the pay period.

Prepare Cathy Wright's payroll check below.

| PERIOD ENDING | EARNINGS | | | DEDUCTIONS | | | | | | | | | NET PAY |
|---|---|---|---|---|---|---|---|---|---|---|---|---|---|
| HOURS WORKED<br>REG.     OT | REGULAR | OVERTIME | TOTAL | FEDERAL INCOME TAX | FICA TAX | STATE INCOME TAX | SDI TAX | HEALTH INS. | SAVINGS | MEDICARE | MISC DED. | TOTAL DED. | AMOUNT |
|  |  |  |  |  |  |  |  |  |  |  |  |  |  |

CHECK # 173977                                                    **Employee:**

---

MOUNTAIN VIEW CLINIC                                             173977
4412 Broadway
London, XY 55555
                                                                 94-72/1224
                              Date: _____

Pay to the order of: _____

_____ Dollars  $ [          ]

Clarion National Bank
          *Member FDIC*
90 Grape Vine Road                    _____
London, XY 55555-0001                      *Authorized Signature*


‖⬛ 005503 ‖⬛ 46782011 ‖⬛ 678800470

2.  Prepare Susan Bronski's payroll check below.

| PERIOD ENDING | EARNINGS | | | DEDUCTIONS | | | | | | | | | NET PAY |
| HOURS WORKED REG.        OT | REGULAR | OVERTIME | TOTAL | FEDERAL INCOME TAX | FICA TAX | STATE INCOME TAX | SDI TAX | HEALTH INS. | SAVINGS | MEDICARE | MISC DED. | TOTAL DED. | AMOUNT |
| | | | | | | | | | | | | | |

CHECK #173978                                                                 **Employee:**

MOUNTAIN VIEW CLINIC                                                      173978
4412 Broadway
London, XY 55555                                          94-72/1224
                                            *Date:* _____

*Pay to the order of:* _____

_____ *Dollars*  $ [            ]

Clarion National Bank
        *Member FDIC*
90 Grape Vine Road                          _____
London, XY 55555-0001                            *Authorized Signature*


||* 005503 ||* 446782011 ||* 678800470

Notes:

Notes:

Notes:

Notes:

Notes:

Notes:

Notes:

Notes: